CHRRONIC PAN

DIET COOKBOOK

The ultimate guide to manage and

Reduce Inflammation with Delicious

Recipes and Day-by-Day Meal Plans

DREW DORSEY

Content

Introduction to Chronic Pancreatitis 7

Role of Nutrition in Managing Chronic Pancreatitis 13

Essential Nutritional Guidelines for Chronic Pancreatitis 17

Pancreatitis-Friendly Recipes 23

Substitutions for Low-Fat Cooking 149

Effective Meal Planning Strategies for Pancreatitis Diet Success 155

"Welcome to a flavorful adventure through balanced culinary delights!"

Introduction to Chronic Pancreatitis

Imagine your pancreas as a tiny factory, churning out digestive enzymes to break down your food. Now, picture that factory under siege, inflamed and struggling to keep up. This is the reality for people living with chronic pancreatitis, a condition where the pancreas becomes permanently damaged.

But fear not! Just like a skilled engineer can reroute production lines, you can learn to manage chronic pancreatitis through dietary adjustments. This guide will be your roadmap to navigating this condition. We'll delve into the science behind chronic pancreatitis, understand how food impacts your inflamed pancreas, and most importantly, equip you with delicious recipes and strategies to build a personalized "pancreatitis-friendly" diet.

This journey starts with understanding the fire within – the causes and symptoms of chronic pancreatitis. We'll then explore the powerful link between what you eat and how your pancreas feels. You'll learn which foods act as allies, aiding digestion, and which ones can stoke the flames of discomfort.

Yet like with a recipe lacking any components, knowledge without action is useless. We'll equip you with the tools to translate this knowledge into delicious and satisfying meals. We'll explore portion control, meal frequency, and low-fat cooking techniques to transform healthy eating into a culinary adventure.

This journey doesn't end in the kitchen. We'll explore how lifestyle modifications and managing stress can further support your well-being. Together, we'll turn the fight against chronic pancreatitis into a delicious and empowering experience.

Understanding Chronic Pancreatitis:

More Than Just a Grumbling Stomach

Have you ever experienced a gnawing pain in your upper abdomen that just will not quit? It might leave you doubled over, reaching for the nearest heating pad. If this sounds familiar, you might be dealing with chronic pancreatitis.

Imagine your pancreas as a tiny, but mighty, organ tucked behind your stomach. It's responsible for two crucial jobs: churning out digestive enzymes to break down your food and producing hormones that regulate your blood sugar. Now, picture this: chronic pancreatitis is like a malfunction in that factory. The pancreas becomes inflamed, leading to long-term damage and a struggle to perform its duties.

This inflammation can trigger a cascade of unpleasant symptoms. The pain in your upper abdomen is a common culprit, often radiating to your back. You might also experience nausea, vomiting, and even weight loss because your body isn't properly absorbing nutrients.

Food as Medicine: Your Diet is Your Ally

Here's where things get interesting. Did you know that what you eat plays a critical role in managing chronic pancreatitis? Think of your diet as a conversation with your pancreas. Certain meals have the potential to aggravate existing inflammation and cause flare-ups. Others, however, can become your allies, easing discomfort and supporting overall health.

This is where the magic of dietary management comes in. By understanding how specific foods affect your pancreas, you can create a personalized "pancreatitis-friendly" diet. It's not about deprivation – it's about empowerment. You'll learn to identify ingredients that work best for you, ensuring you get the essential nutrients your body needs without the discomfort.

This Cookbook: Your Culinary Compass on the Road to Relief

This cookbook is more than just a collection of recipes; it's your guide to navigating the world of chronic pancreatitis with delicious confidence.

Inside, you'll find:

Clear explanations: We'll break down the science behind chronic pancreatitis and dietary management in a way that's easy to understand.

Food friends and foes: You'll discover which foods can aggravate your symptoms and which ones can act as allies, promoting better digestion and overall well-being.

Delicious recipes: Forget bland and boring! We offer a variety of mouthwatering dishes that are not only tasty but also specifically tailored for a pancreatitis-friendly diet. From protein-packed breakfasts to satisfying dinners, you'll find something to tantalize your taste buds at every meal.

Cooking techniques for success: We'll share low-fat cooking methods and strategies that make healthy eating enjoyable and effortless.

This cookbook is your partner on the path to managing chronic pancreatitis. Together, we'll transform your diet from a source of frustration into a tool for reclaiming your health and enjoying delicious food along the way. Remember, you're not alone in this journey. Let this book be your culinary compass, guiding you towards a life filled with flavor and well-being.

Role of Nutrition in Managing Chronic Pancreatitis

Nutritional Impact on Pancreatitis

Chronic pancreatitis throws a wrench into your digestive system. Your inflamed pancreas struggles to produce the enzymes needed to break down food, especially fats and proteins. This can lead to a domino effect on your overall health.

Here is how your diet directly impacts your pancreas:

Fat Overload: Fats are the primary fuel source for your body, but they also require the most work for your pancreas to break down. When you consume too much fat, your pancreas gets overwhelmed. This can worsen inflammation and trigger painful flares.

Protein Power Struggle: Protein is another crucial building block for your body, but digesting it also puts a strain on your pancreas. Undigested protein fragments can irritate the inflamed tissue, causing discomfort.

Micronutrient Mishap: When your pancreas isn't functioning optimally, your body might struggle to absorb essential vitamins and minerals from food. This can lead to deficiencies that impact your overall health and well-being.

Dietary Factors: Turning Down the Heat on Pancreatitis

Now that you understand the impact of food on your pancreas, let us explore specific dietary factors that can influence your symptoms:

Fats: Limiting saturated and unhealthy fats, found in fried foods, fatty meats, and processed snacks, is key. These fats are difficult to digest and can exacerbate inflammation. Instead, focus on "good fats" like those found in fish, avocados, and nuts, which are easier for your pancreas to manage.

Protein Power: opt for lean protein sources like skinless chicken, fish, and beans. These options are easier on your digestive system and provide essential amino acids for your body. Limiting red meat and processed meats can further reduce stress on your pancreas.

Sugar Rush: Simple sugars found in candy, sugary drinks, and refined carbohydrates can cause blood sugar spikes. This puts a strain on your pancreas, which also produces insulin to regulate blood sugar. Choosing complex carbohydrates from fruits, vegetables, and whole grains provides sustained energy without the sugar rush.

Fiber Friend: Fiber plays a crucial role in digestion. It helps move food through your system smoothly and can even promote satiety, keeping you feeling fuller for longer. opt for fruits, vegetables, and whole grains rich in fiber to support your digestive system.

Alcohol Abuse: Alcohol is a significant risk factor for chronic pancreatitis. It can directly damage pancreatic tissue and worsen inflammation. Eliminating alcohol consumption is highly recommended for managing symptoms.

The Power of a Pancreatitis-Focused Diet: Beyond Symptom Relief

By following a pancreatitis-focused diet, you'll experience benefits that extend far beyond simply managing pain. *Here is what you can expect:*

Reduced Flares: By minimizing the intake of foods that trigger inflammation, you can significantly reduce the frequency and intensity of painful flares. This translates to a better quality of life with less discomfort.

Improved Nutrient Absorption: With a diet tailored for your pancreas, your body becomes more efficient at absorbing essential nutrients from food. This translates to better overall health and increased energy levels.

Weight Management: Chronic pancreatitis can sometimes lead to weight loss due to malabsorption. A balanced pancreatitis-friendly diet helps you maintain a healthy weight by providing adequate nutrition without overloading your digestive system.

Empowerment: Taking control of your diet through this approach empowers you to actively manage your chronic pancreatitis. This sense of control can significantly improve your well-being and overall outlook on your health.

Essential Nutritional Guidelines for Chronic Pancreatitis

Mastering the Macronutrients: Fueling Your Body for Pancreatitis Wellness

When it comes to managing chronic pancreatitis, understanding macronutrients—fats, proteins, and carbohydrates—becomes crucial. Here's a breakdown of how each plays a role in your health and specific recommendations for a pancreatitis-friendly diet:

Fats:

Remember, fat is the primary culprit that can overwhelm your pancreas. *Here is the key:*

- *Limit Saturated and Unsaturated Fats*: Minimize saturated fats found in fatty meats, fried foods, and processed snacks. These are the most challenging for your pancreas to digest. Limit unhealthy unsaturated fats, like those in processed vegetable oils and baked goods.

- **Embrace "Good Fats":** Focus on including healthy monounsaturated and polyunsaturated fats, found in:
- **Fish:** Salmon, tuna, and sardines are excellent sources of omega-3 fatty acids, which offer anti-inflammatory benefits.
- **Avocados:** These creamy fruits are packed with healthy fats and essential vitamins.
- **Nuts and Seeds:** Rich sources of fiber and healthy fats include almonds, walnuts, flaxseeds, and chia seeds.

Protein:

Protein is essential for building and repairing tissues. However, your pancreas needs to work hard to break it down. *Here is how to strike a balance:*

- **Choose lean protein sources:** opt for protein sources that are easier to digest, such as:

- ***Skinless Chicken and Turkey:*** These are classic lean protein options that are versatile for various dishes.

- ***Fish:*** As mentioned earlier, fish offers protein along with healthy fats.

- ***Beans and legumes:*** These plant-based protein sources are packed with fiber as well.

- ***Moderate Protein Intake:*** While protein is crucial, excessive amounts can put a strain on your pancreas. Talk to your doctor or a registered dietitian to determine the appropriate protein intake for you.

Carbohydrates:

Carbohydrates provide your body with energy. However, refined carbohydrates can cause blood sugar spikes, stressing your pancreas. ***Here is what to prioritize:***

- ***Focus on Complex Carbs:*** Choose complex carbohydrates found in:

- *Fruits and vegetables:* These offer essential vitamins, minerals, and fiber alongside natural sugars.
- *Whole Grains:* Brown rice, quinoa, and whole-wheat bread provide sustained energy without the sugar rush.
- *Limit Simple Sugars:* Minimize refined carbohydrates like sugary drinks, white bread, and pastries.

Essential Vitamins and Minerals:

While macronutrients provide the bulk of your energy, vitamins and minerals play a crucial role in overall health, including pancreatic function. *Here are some key players:*

- *Fat-Soluble Vitamins (A, D, E, and K):* Since fat absorption might be an issue, talk to your doctor about supplements to ensure you get enough of these crucial vitamins.
- *Vitamin B Complex:* These vitamins play a role in various bodily functions, including enzyme production. Reliable sources include

leafy green vegetables, beans, and whole grains.

- *Vitamin C:* This powerful antioxidant helps reduce inflammation and supports immunity. Vitamin C is abundant in fruits and vegetables.

- *Calcium:* This mineral is essential for strong bones and may also play a role in pancreatic function. Dairy products (if tolerated) and leafy green vegetables are thorough sources.

Portion Control and Meal Frequency for Pancreatitis

Portion control and meal frequency work together to manage your chronic pancreatitis:

Portion Control:

- *Think Smaller Plates:* Using smaller plates can create a feeling of fullness with less food, helping you avoid overeating and overwhelming your pancreas.

- *Focus on Quality, Not Quantity:* Prioritize nutrient-dense foods so you get the most out of each bite.
- *Listen to your body:* Pay attention to hunger cues and avoid overstuffing yourself. Once you're satisfied, stop eating.

Meal Frequency:

- *Smaller, More Frequent Meals:* Instead of three large meals, aim for 5–6 smaller meals and snacks throughout the day. This keeps your digestive system working consistently and reduces the workload on your pancreas at any given time.
- *Plan Your Meals:* Having a plan helps you make healthy choices and avoid impulsive snacking.
- *Do not Skip Meals:* Skipping meals can trigger pain. Make every effort to adhere to the timetable you have set up.

By following these guidelines and the personalized recommendations from your healthcare team, you can create a sustainable and effective dietary approach to manage your chronic pancreatitis.

Pancreatitis-Friendly Recipes

Breakfast recipes

High-Protein Smoothie

Ingredients:

- 1 cup low-fat milk (dairy or plant-based)
- ½ cup low-fat Greek yogurt
- 1 scoop protein powder (approved by your doctor)
- 1 cup spinach, fresh or frozen
- ½ cup frozen berries
- ¼ cup chopped banana (optional)
- ¼ teaspoon ground cinnamon (optional)

Instructions:

- Add all the ingredients to a blender.
- Scrape down the sides as necessary, and blend until creamy and smooth.
- Enjoy immediately!

Total Preparation Time: 5 minutes

Servings: 1

Nutritional Information (approximate values per serving):
Calories: 300–400 (depending on protein powder)
Protein: 20–30 grams (depending on protein powder)
Carbohydrates: 30–40 grams
Fat: 5–10 grams

Tips:

- Adjust the protein powder amount based on your doctor's recommendations.
- Substitute berries with other frozen fruits like mango, pineapple, or peaches.
- Add a drizzle of honey or maple syrup for extra sweetness (use sparingly).
- Use nut butter (almond or peanut butter) for a thicker and creamier texture (moderation due to calorie content).

- For a thicker consistency, add a few ice cubes.
- Blend with a handful of chopped kale or other leafy greens for an extra nutrient boost.

Tofu Scramble with Türkiye Sausage

Ingredients:

- One 14-oz block of firm tofu that has been drained and pressed.
- 4 oz. ground turkey sausage
- ½ cup chopped onion
- ½ cup chopped bell pepper (any color)
- ¼ cup chopped mushrooms (optional)
- 1 clove garlic, minced
- ½ teaspoon turmeric powder
- ¼ teaspoon smoked paprika
- ¼ teaspoon black pepper
- ¼ cup chopped fresh parsley (optional)
- 2 tablespoons olive oil
- Salt to taste
- ¼ cup low-fat shredded cheese (optional)

- Whole-wheat toast or tortillas (for serving)

Instructions:

- Crumble the tofu with your hands or a fork in a bowl.
- In a big skillet over medium heat, warm up the olive oil. After adding, simmer for approximately 5 minutes, or until the peppers and onions are tender.
- Add the ground turkey sausage and cook until browned, breaking it up with a spoon.
- Stir in the garlic, turmeric, paprika, and black pepper. Cook until aromatic, about 1 more minute.
- Add the crumbled tofu to the skillet and cook for a few minutes, stirring occasionally, to allow the tofu to absorb the flavors.
- Season with salt to taste. (Be mindful if using pre-seasoned sausage.)
- Stir in chopped fresh parsley (optional) and cook for another minute.

- Serve immediately over whole-wheat toast or tortillas. Top with shredded cheese (optional).

Cooking Time: 15 minutes

Total Preparation Time: 20 minutes

Servings: two

Nutritional Information (approximate values per serving, without cheese):
Calories: 350-400
Protein: 30-35 grams
Carbohydrates: 20-25 grams
Fat: 15-20 grams

Tips:

- Freeze leftover crumbled tofu for future use in scrambles.
- Add other chopped vegetables, like broccoli or zucchini to the scramble.
- Use vegan cheese or omit cheese altogether for a dairy-free option.
- For a spicier scramble, add a pinch of red pepper flakes.

- Serve with a side of salsa or avocado slices (moderation) for added flavor and healthy fats.

Egg White Frittata with Vegetables

Ingredients:

- Four egg whites
- 1/2 cup chopped vegetables (broccoli, bell peppers, onions - your choice)
- 1/4 cup shredded low-fat cheese (optional)
- 1 tablespoon olive oil
- Salt and pepper to taste
- Fresh herbs (optional)

Instructions:

- Preheat oven to 375°F (190°C). Lightly grease a non-stick oven-safe skillet.
- Beat the egg whites with a fork until foamy. Season with salt and pepper.
- Heat olive oil in the preheated skillet over medium heat. Add chopped vegetables and cook until softened, about 5 minutes.

- Pour the egg white mixture over the vegetables in the skillet.
- Sprinkle shredded cheese on top (if using).
- Bake for 20-25 minutes, or until the center is set and the top is lightly golden brown.
- Serve right away after adding a fresh herb garnish (optional).

Cooking Time: 20-25 minutes

Total Preparation Time: 30 minutes

Servings: 2-3

Nutritional Information (per serving, without cheese):
Calories: 140
Protein: 12g
Carbohydrates: 5g
Fat: 7g

Tips:

- Get creative with your vegetables! You can use spinach, mushrooms, asparagus, or any other favorites.
- For a vegetarian option, omit the cheese.

- You may reheat leftovers in the microwave after storing them in the refrigerator for up

Chicken Sausage and Veggie Muffins

Ingredients:

- 1 pound cooked and crumbled chicken sausage
- 1 cup chopped vegetables (broccoli, bell peppers, onions - your choice)
- 1/2 cup chopped whole-wheat bread (toasted and crumbled)
- 1/4 cup low-fat milk
- 2 large eggs
- 1/4 cup shredded low-fat cheese (optional)
- Salt and pepper to taste

Instructions:

- Preheat oven to 375°F (190°C). Grease a 12-cup muffin tin.
- In a large bowl, combine cooked chicken sausage, chopped vegetables, and crumbled whole-wheat bread.

- Whisk the eggs and milk together in another basin. Sprinkle some salt and pepper on it.
- Transfer the egg mixture into the bowl containing the vegetable mixture, chicken sausage, and sausage. Toss to blend.
- Evenly divide the mixture among the muffin cups that have been prepared.
- Add shredded cheese on top, if using.
- A toothpick inserted in the center should come out clean after 20 to 25 minutes of baking, or until the muffins are golden brown.
- Before taking them out of the muffin tray, allow them to cool slightly.

Cooking Time: 20-25 minutes

Total Preparation Time: 30 minutes

Servings: 12 muffins

Nutritional Information (per muffin, without cheese):
Calories: 180
Protein: 10g

Carbohydrates: 15g
Fat: 8g

Tips:

- You can use pre-cooked chicken sausage for convenience.
- Experiment with different types of vegetables and cheeses.
- You may freeze these muffins for up to three months. Reheat in the microwave before serving.

Greek Yogurt Parfait with Nuts and Seeds

Ingredients:

- 1 cup low-fat Greek yogurt
- 1/2 cup sliced fruit (berries, banana, mango - your choice)
- 1/4 cup chopped nuts and seeds (almonds, walnuts, chia seeds - choose a combination)
- 1 tablespoon honey (optional)
- A sprinkle of granola (optional)

Instructions:

- In a serving glass or bowl, layer the Greek yogurt, sliced fruit, and chopped nuts and seeds.
- Drizzle with honey (if using) and sprinkle with granola (if using).

Total Preparation Time: 5 minutes

Servings: 1

Nutritional Information (per serving, with honey and granola):
Calories: 300
Protein: 20g
Carbohydrates: 35g
Fat: 8g

<u>Tips:</u>

- Use any type of fruit you like. Frozen fruit can be used as well, just thaw slightly before assembling the parfait.
- For a vegan option, use plant-based yogurt.
- You can adjust the amount of honey and granola to your taste preference.

<u>High-Protein Oatmeal with Berries</u>

Ingredients:

- 1/2 cup rolled oats
- 1 cup low-fat milk
- 1/2 cup water
- 1 scoop protein powder (approved by your doctor)
- 1/4 cup fresh or frozen berries
- 1/4 teaspoon ground cinnamon
- Pinch of salt (optional)

Instructions:

- In a saucepan, combine oats, milk, water, protein powder, and cinnamon.
- Over medium heat, bring to a boil while stirring from time to time.
- Reduce heat to low and simmer for 5 minutes, or until oats are cooked through and desired consistency is reached (add more water if needed for a creamier texture).
- Remove from heat and stir in berries.

Cooking Time: 5 minutes

Total Preparation Time: 10 minutes

Servings: 1

Nutritional Information (approximate):
Calories: 300
Protein: 20g
Carbohydrates: 40g
Fat: 5g

Tips:

- Use a variety of berries for extra flavor and nutrients.
- Top with a sprinkle of chopped nuts or seeds for added protein and healthy fats.
- Sweeten with a drizzle of honey or maple syrup (use sparingly).
- For a thicker oatmeal, use less water or cook for a longer time.

Türkiye Bacon and Whole-Wheat Pancakes

Ingredients:

- One cup whole-wheat flour
- One teaspoon baking powder
- 1/4 teaspoon baking soda
- 1/4 teaspoon salt

- 1 cup low-fat milk
- 1 egg white
- 1 tablespoon melted low-fat butter or oil.
- Two slices cooked turkey bacon, crumbled.
- Cooking spray

Instructions:

- Mix the flour, baking soda, baking powder, and salt in a medium-sized basin.
- Mix the melted butter, egg white, and milk in another basin.
- A few lumps are OK when folding the wet components into the dry ingredients until they are just mixed. Avoid over-mixing.
- Heat a skillet or griddle that has been gently oiled over medium heat.
- Spray a non-stick pan with cooking spray and pour 1/4 cup of batter per pancake.
- Sprinkle crumbled turkey bacon on top of each pancake batter.
- Cook for 2 to 3 minutes on each side, or until well cooked and golden brown.
- Flip pancakes carefully using a spatula.

Cooking Time: 2-3 minutes per side

Total Preparation Time: 15 minutes

Servings: 2-3 pancakes

Nutritional Information (approximate per pancake):
Calories: 150
Protein: 10g
Carbohydrates: 20g
Fat: 5g

Tips:

- Replace turkey bacon with chopped cooked chicken sausage for a different flavor.
- Add a handful of blueberries or chopped nuts to the batter for extra flavor and nutrients.
- Serve with a dollop of low-fat yogurt and a drizzle of sugar-free maple syrup.
- Leftover cooked pancakes can be stored in the refrigerator for up to 3 days and reheated in a toaster oven.

Lentil Soup with Cottage Cheese

Ingredients:

- One cup dried brown lentil, rinsed.
- Four cups low-sodium vegetable broth
- One tablespoon olive oil
- One onion, chopped.
- Two carrots, chopped.
- Two celery stalks, chopped.
- 2 cloves garlic, minced.
- One teaspoon dried thyme
- 1/2 teaspoon ground cumin
- 1 (14.5 oz) can diced tomatoes, undrained
- Salt and black pepper to taste
- One cup low-fat cottage cheese
- Chopped fresh parsley (optional, for garnish)

Instructions:

- Warm up the olive oil in a big saucepan over medium heat. Add the celery, carrots, and onion. Sauté until softened, about 5 minutes.
- Stir in cumin, thyme, and garlic. Cook, stirring regularly, for one more minute.

- Add the chopped tomatoes, vegetable broth, and rinsed lentils. Once the lentils are cooked, simmer for 20 to 25 minutes on low heat after bringing to a boil.
- Season with salt and pepper to taste.
- Once lentils are cooked, ladle soup into bowls. Top with a dollop of cottage cheese and garnish with chopped fresh parsley (optional).

Cooking Time: 25 minutes

Total Preparation Time: 30 minutes

Servings: 4

Nutritional Information (per serving):
Calories: 280
Protein: 18g
Carbohydrates: 40g
Fat: 7g

Tips:

- For a thicker soup, mash some of the cooked lentils against the side of the pot with a fork before adding the cottage cheese.

- You can substitute green lentils for brown lentils in this recipe.
- Add a splash of lemon juice or a sprinkle of red pepper flakes for extra flavor.
- You may keep leftovers in the fridge for up to three days if you put them in an airtight container.

Scrambled Eggs with Black Beans and Salsa

Ingredients:

- Two large eggs
- One egg white (optional, for extra protein)
- 1 tablespoon low-fat milk
- 1/4 cup cooked black beans, rinsed, and drained.
- 1/4 cup chopped tomatoes.
- 1/4 cup chopped red onion.
- 1/4 cup salsa (choose your preferred level of spiciness)
- 1/2 teaspoon olive oil
- Salt and black pepper to taste

- Chopped fresh cilantro (optional, for garnish)

Instructions:

- In a bowl, whisk together eggs, egg white (if using), and milk. Season with salt and pepper.
- In a nonstick pan, warm the olive oil over medium heat. Cook the chopped onion for two to three minutes, or until it becomes tender.
- To the pan, add the diced tomatoes and black beans. Stirring occasionally, cook for one more minute. Pour in the egg mixture and scramble continuously with a spatula until the eggs are cooked through to the desired consistency.
- Remove from heat and stir in salsa.
- Serve immediately on a plate. Garnish with chopped fresh cilantro (optional).

Cooking Time: 5-7 minutes

Total Preparation Time: 10 minutes

Servings: 1

Nutritional Information (per serving):
Calories: 250
Protein: 18g
Carbohydrates: 15g
Fat: 7g

Tips:

- For simpler cleanup and to avoid sticking, use a non-stick pan.

- If you prefer a creamier texture, you can add a tablespoon of low-fat cottage cheese to the egg mixture before scrambling.

- You can use canned black beans for convenience, just be sure to rinse and drain them well.

- Feel free to adjust the amount of salsa to your desired level of spiciness.

- Leftovers can be stored in an airtight container in the refrigerator for up to 1 day. Reheat gently over low heat.

High-Protein Smoothie Bowl

Ingredients:

- One cup unsweetened almond milk (or low-fat milk)
- 1/2 cup frozen mixed berries
- One-half banana (frozen or fresh)
- One scoop protein powder (approved by your doctor)
- One tablespoon chia seeds
- 1/4 cup chopped nuts and seeds (almonds, walnuts, flaxseeds) - for garnish (optional)
- Fresh fruit slices (banana, kiwi, strawberries) - for garnish (optional)

Instructions:

- Prep (2 minutes): Gather all ingredients and pre-portion toppings like nuts and fruits. If using fresh banana, slice it.
- Blend (2 minutes): Combine almond milk, frozen berries, banana, protein powder, and chia seeds in a blender. Blend until smooth and creamy.
- Assemble (1 minute): Pour the smoothie mixture into a bowl.

- Garnish (1 minute): Top with chopped nuts and seeds, fresh fruit slices, or a drizzle of honey (optional).

Total Preparation Time: 6 minutes

Serving Size: 1

Nutritional Information (approximate):
Calories: 350-400
Protein: 20-25 grams
Carbohydrates: 40-50 grams
Fat: 5-10 grams (depending on nut/seed toppings)

Tips:

- You may adjust the thickness of the smoothie by adding milk.
- Substitute frozen berries with other frozen fruits like mango, pineapple, or peaches.
- Use a protein powder with natural flavors or add a touch of cinnamon or vanilla extract for extra flavor.
- For a thicker base, add a tablespoon of rolled oats or nut butter (approved by your doctor) to the blender.

- Freeze leftover smoothie portions in single-serve containers for a quick and easy breakfast or snack later.

Brunch recipes.

<u>Türkiye and Veggie Frittata</u>

Ingredients:

- Six egg whites
- 1/4 cup chopped onion.
- 1/2 cup chopped bell peppers (any color)
- 1/2 cup chopped broccoli florets.
- 1/2 cup chopped spinach.
- 1 cup cooked, shredded turkey breast.
- 1/4 cup crumbled low-fat feta cheese (optional)
- 1 tablespoon olive oil
- Salt and pepper to taste

Instructions:

- Preheat oven to 375°F (190°C). Grease a 9-inch ovenproof skillet with cooking spray.

- In a large skillet, heat the olive oil over medium heat. Add the onions and simmer for approximately 3 minutes, or until softened.
- Add bell peppers and broccoli, cook for another 2-3 minutes until slightly tender-crisp.
- In a large bowl, whisk together egg whites, salt, and pepper. Stir in cooked vegetables, spinach, and shredded turkey.
- Pour the egg mixture into the preheated skillet. If using feta cheese, sprinkle evenly over the top.
- Bake for 20-25 minutes, or until the middle is firm and a toothpick inserted comes out clean.
- Allow to cool slightly before cutting into wedges and serving.

Cooking Time: 20-25 minutes

Total Preparation Time: 30 minutes

Servings: 4

Nutritional Information (per serving):

Calories: 250
Protein: 25g
Carbohydrates: 10g
Fat: 12g (including healthy fats from olive oil)

Tips:

- Add other chopped vegetables like mushrooms, zucchini, or cherry tomatoes for additional flavor and texture.
- If you prefer a firmer frittata, pre-cook the turkey breast in a separate pan and add it to the egg mixture along with the vegetables.
- For a vegetarian option, omit the turkey and add another 1/2 cup of cooked chopped vegetables.
- Refrigerate leftovers in an airtight jar for up to three days.

Shrimp and Quinoa Salad with Avocado

Ingredients:

- One cup cooked quinoa
- 1-pound cooked, peeled shrimp (deveined and tails removed)

- 1 cup chopped celery.
- 1/2 cup chopped cucumber.
- 1/4 cup chopped red onion.
- 1/4 cup chopped fresh parsley.
- One avocado, diced (use sparingly)
- Three tablespoons olive oil
- Two tablespoons lemon juice
- One tablespoon Dijon mustard
- Salt and pepper to taste

Instructions:

- In a large bowl, combine cooked quinoa, shrimp, celery, cucumber, red onion, and parsley.
- In a separate bowl, combine the olive oil, lemon juice, Dijon mustard, salt, and pepper.
- Pour the dressing over the salad ingredients and toss to cover evenly.
- Gently fold in the diced avocado just before serving.

Cooking Time: N/A (depends on cooking method for quinoa and shrimp)

Total Preparation Time: 20 minutes (assuming quinoa and shrimp are already cooked)

Servings: 4

Nutritional Information (per serving):
Calories: 400
Protein: 30g
Carbohydrates: 40g
Fat: 15g (including healthy fats from avocado and olive oil)

Tips:

- Use leftover cooked quinoa or shrimp to save time.
- You can substitute other vegetables like chopped bell peppers, cherry tomatoes, or corn.
- For a creamier dressing, add a dollop of low-fat Greek yogurt.
- Serve the salad on a bed of lettuce for a more filling meal.

Salmon with Roasted Sweet Potatoes and Asparagus

Ingredients:

- Two salmon fillets (6 oz each)
- One tablespoon olive oil
- 1/2 teaspoon dried dill
- 1/4 teaspoon salt
- 1/4 teaspoon black pepper
- One medium sweet potato, around one cup, peeled and chopped.
- One bunch asparagus, trimmed.
- One tablespoon lemon juice (optional)

Instructions:

- Preheat oven to 400°F (200°C). Line a baking sheet with parchment paper.
- In a small bowl, combine olive oil, dill, salt, and pepper. Apply the mixture to the salmon fillets.
- Place the salmon fillets on the prepared baking sheet.
- Toss the diced sweet potato with a drizzle of olive oil and a pinch of salt and pepper. Spread the sweet potato cubes around the salmon on the baking sheet.

- Trim the asparagus ends and toss with a drizzle of olive oil and a pinch of salt and pepper. Arrange the asparagus spears next to the salmon and sweet potatoes.
- Bake for 15-20 minutes, or until the salmon is cooked through (flaky with a fork) and the vegetables are tender-crisp.
- (Optional) Squeeze some fresh lemon juice over the salmon before serving.

Cooking Time: 15-20 minutes

Total Preparation Time: 20-25 minutes

Servings: 2

Nutritional Information (per serving):
Calories: 450-500
Protein: 30-35 grams
Carbohydrates: 30-35 grams
Fat: 20-25 grams

Tips:

- You can substitute other herbs for dill, such as rosemary or thyme.

- For a vegetarian option, replace the salmon with tofu cubes marinated in a similar sauce.
- Add a side salad with a light vinaigrette dressing for a more complete meal.

Tofu Scramble Breakfast Burrito

Ingredients:

- One 14-oz block of firm tofu that has been drained and pressed.
- One tablespoon olive oil
- One-half onion, diced.
- One bell pepper (any color), diced.
- 1/2 cup chopped mushrooms (optional)
- 1/4 teaspoon turmeric
- 1/4 teaspoon smoked paprika.
- 1/4 teaspoon chili powder (optional)
- Salt and black pepper to taste
- 2 large whole-wheat tortillas
- 1/4 cup shredded low-fat cheddar cheese (optional)
- 1/4 cup chopped fresh salsa.
- 1/4 cup chopped avocado (optional)

Instructions:

- Use a fork or your hands to crumble the tofu.

- In a skillet set over medium heat, warm the olive oil. After adding the onion, heat for about five minutes, or until it becomes soft.

- Add the bell pepper and mushrooms (if using) and cook for another 5 minutes, or until softened.

- Stir in the crumbled tofu, turmeric, paprika, chili powder (if using), salt, and pepper. Cook the tofu for a few minutes, or until it is well heated.

- The whole-wheat tortillas can be briefly warmed in the microwave or a dry pan.

- Spread the tofu scramble evenly down the center of each tortilla.

- Top with shredded cheese (if using), salsa, and avocado (if using).

- Fold the bottom of the tortilla up and over the filling, then fold in the sides and roll up tightly.

Cooking Time: 15-20 minutes

Total Preparation Time: 20-25 minutes

Servings: two

Nutritional Information (per serving, without cheese and avocado):
Calories: 350-400
Protein: 20-25 grams
Carbohydrates: 30-35 grams
Fat: 15-20 grams

Tips:

- You can add other vegetables to the scramble, such as chopped spinach, broccoli, or tomatoes.
- Use a vegan cheese alternative if you prefer a dairy-free option.
- Serve the burritos with a side of fruit salad or yogurt for a balanced breakfast.

Chicken Breast with Whole-Wheat Pancakes and Berries

Ingredients:

For the Chicken:

- One boneless, skinless chicken breast (around 150g)
- 1/2 tablespoon olive oil
- Salt and pepper to taste
- For the Whole-Wheat Pancakes:
- One cup whole-wheat flour
- One teaspoon baking powder
- 1/4 teaspoon baking soda
- 1/4 teaspoon salt
- One cup low-fat milk
- One large egg
- One tablespoon melted butter (or a light cooking spray)

For the Berries:

- One cup of berries, either fresh or frozen (strawberries, raspberries, and blueberries)
- One tablespoon maple syrup (optional)

Instructions:

Prepare the Chicken (Cook Time: 15-20 minutes, Prep Time: 5 minutes):

- Heat up a skillet or grill pan to a medium temperature.
- Season the chicken breast with salt and pepper.
- Add olive oil to the pan and cook the chicken breast for 7-8 minutes per side, or until cooked through (internal temperature reaches 165°F).
- Remove from heat and let rest for a few minutes before slicing.

Prepare the Whole-Wheat Pancakes (Cook Time: 5 minutes per pancake, Prep Time: 5 minutes):

- In a large bowl, whisk together the whole-wheat flour, baking powder, baking soda, and salt.
- In a separate bowl, whisk together the milk, egg, and melted butter (or use cooking spray to coat a pan).
- Combine the wet and dry ingredients until just combined (a few lumps are okay).
- Heat a griddle or pan that has been gently oiled over medium heat.

- For each pancake, transfer 1/4 cup of batter to the skillet.
- Cook for two to three minutes on each side, or until the edges begin to firm and bubbles form on the surface. After one or two more minutes, flip and continue cooking until golden brown.

Assemble and Serve:

- Plate the sliced chicken breast alongside 2-3 whole-wheat pancakes.
- Top the pancakes with fresh or frozen berries.
- Drizzle with maple syrup (optional) and enjoy!

Total Preparation Time: 25-30 minutes

Servings: 1

Nutritional Information (approximate values per serving):
Calories: 450-500
Protein: 40-45g
Carbohydrates: 50-55g

Fat: 15-20g

Tips:

- You can marinate the chicken breast in a low-fat marinade for additional flavor before cooking.

- Reduce the amount of milk in the batter slightly to get thicker pancakes.

- For more sweetness, try substituting some honey or low-sugar fruit compote for the maple syrup.

- You may keep leftover chicken in the fridge for up to three days if you put it in an airtight container. Reheat gently before serving.

- Add a side of low-fat yogurt or cottage cheese for an extra protein boost.

Lunch recipes.

Chicken Caesar Salad with Grilled Chicken Breast, Protein Powder

Ingredients:

For the Chicken:

- 1 boneless, skinless chicken breast (around 150g)
- 1 tablespoon olive oil
- 1/2 teaspoon dried oregano
- 1/4 teaspoon garlic powder
- Salt and black pepper to taste

For the Salad:

- 2 cups romaine lettuce, chopped.
- 1/2 cup cherry tomatoes, halved.
- 1/4 cup grated Parmesan cheese (optional)
- 2 tablespoons croutons (whole-wheat preferred)

For the Dressing:

- 2 tablespoons low-fat Caesar dressing
- 1/2 scoop protein powder (approved by your doctor)
- 1 tablespoon lemon juice
- 1 tablespoon freshly grated Parmesan cheese (optional)

Instructions:

- Marinate the Chicken (15 minutes): In a bowl, combine olive oil, oregano, garlic powder, salt, and pepper. Add the chicken breast and toss to coat. For maximum taste, marinate for up to 30 minutes, but at least 15 minutes is plenty.
- Grill the Chicken (10-12 minutes): Preheat your grill to medium-high heat. Grill the chicken breast for 10-12 minutes per side, or until cooked through (internal temperature reaches 165°F). Set aside to cool slightly.
- Prepare the Dressing (5 minutes): In a small bowl, whisk together Caesar dressing, protein powder, lemon juice, and optional Parmesan cheese.
- Assemble the Salad (5 minutes): In a large bowl, combine chopped romaine lettuce, cherry tomatoes, and croutons. Slice the cooled chicken breast and add it to the salad. Drizzle with the prepared Caesar dressing and toss to coat. Garnish with additional Parmesan cheese (optional) and serve.

Total Preparation Time: 30 minutes

Cooking Time: 10-12 minutes (grilling chicken)

Servings: 1

Nutritional Information (approximate per serving):
Calories: 450-500
Protein: 50-55g (depending on protein powder)
Carbohydrates: 30-35g
Fat: 20-25g

Tips:

- You can use leftover grilled chicken for this recipe.

- If you don't have a grill, you can bake the chicken breast at 400°F (200°C) for 20-25 minutes, or until cooked through.

- To suit your taste, make adjustments to the quantity of dressing.

- For a vegan option, omit the Parmesan cheese and use a vegan Caesar dressing.

Lentil and Black Bean Salad with Quinoa

Ingredients:

- 1 cup dry brown lentils, rinsed.
- One can (15 oz) of rinsed and drained black beans
- 1 cup cooked quinoa
- 1 cup chopped vegetables (combination of bell peppers, corn, cucumber, or cherry tomatoes)
- 1/4 cup chopped red onion.
- 1/4 cup chopped fresh cilantro.
- 2 tablespoons olive oil
- 2 tablespoons lemon juice
- 1 tablespoon apple cider vinegar (optional)
- 1 teaspoon ground cumin
- 1/2 teaspoon chili powder
- Salt and black pepper to taste

Instructions:

- In a medium saucepan, cook the lentils according to package instructions. Drain and set aside to cool.
- While the lentils cook, prepare the quinoa according to package instructions and fluff with a fork. Set aside to cool slightly.

- In a large bowl, combine cooled lentils, black beans, quinoa, chopped vegetables, red onion, and cilantro.
- In a small bowl, whisk together olive oil, lemon juice, apple cider vinegar (if using), cumin, chili powder, salt, and pepper.
- Drizzle the salad items with the dressing and gently toss to coat.
- To taste, add more salt and pepper for seasoning.

Cooking Time: Lentil cooking time will vary depending on the type of lentil used (usually 20-30 minutes). Quinoa cooking time will also vary depending on the brand (usually 15-20 minutes).

Total Preparation Time: 30-40 minutes (depending on lentil cooking time)

Servings: 4-6

Nutritional Information (per serving):
Calories: 300-350 (approximate)
Protein: 15-20 grams (approximate)
Carbohydrates: 40-45 grams (approximate)

Fat: 10-12 grams (approximate)

Tips:

- For a vegetarian option, omit the black beans and add another cup of cooked lentils.
- Feel free to adjust the vegetables based on your preferences. Chopped zucchini, chopped carrots, or chopped celery would also work well in this salad.
- For up to three days, leftovers can be kept in the refrigerator in an airtight container.

Turkey Burger on Whole-Wheat Bun with Avocado

Ingredients:

- 1 pound ground turkey breast
- 1/4 cup breadcrumbs
- 1/4 cup chopped onion.
- 1 egg white, lightly beaten
- 1 tablespoon Worcestershire sauce
- 1 teaspoon dried thyme
- 1/2 teaspoon garlic powder
- 1/4 teaspoon salt

- 1/4 teaspoon black pepper
- 1 whole-wheat hamburger bun, toasted
- 1/4 avocado, sliced (optional)
- Lettuce leaves
- Tomato slice (optional)
- Onion slice (optional)
- Low-fat mayonnaise or mustard (optional)

Instructions:

- In a large bowl, combine ground turkey, breadcrumbs, chopped onion, egg white, Worcestershire sauce, thyme, garlic powder, salt, and pepper. Gently blend with your hands until well-integrated.
- Form the mixture into two hamburger patties.
- Heat a large skillet over medium heat. Add a touch of olive oil or cooking spray.
- Cook the burger patties until they are thoroughly cooked, about 4–5 minutes per side.
- While the burgers are cooking, toast the whole-wheat bun.

- Assemble your burger on the toasted bun with lettuce, tomato, onion (if using), avocado slices (optional), and a drizzle of low-fat mayonnaise or mustard (if using).

Cooking Time: 8-10 minutes (4-5 minutes per side)

Total Preparation Time: 15-20 minutes

Servings: 2

Nutritional Information (per serving, without avocado):
Calories: 400-450 (approximate)
Protein: 30-35 grams (approximate)
Carbohydrates: 30-35 grams (approximate)
Fat: 15-20 grams (approximate)

Tips:

- You can add other chopped vegetables to the burger mixture, such as grated carrots or chopped bell peppers.
- If you don't have breadcrumbs, you can crush whole-wheat crackers or tortilla chips.

- To make the burgers lower in fat, drain any excess grease from the pan after cooking.
- To suit your taste, feel free to experiment with the seasonings.

Tuna Salad Sandwich with Cottage Cheese on Whole-Wheat Bread

Ingredients:

- Two slices of whole-wheat bread, toasted.
- 5 oz canned tuna in water, drained.
- 1/4 cup low-fat cottage cheese
- 1 tablespoon light mayonnaise
- 1 stalk celery finely chopped.
- 1/4 red onion finely chopped.
- Pinch of dried dill (optional)
- Salt and black pepper to taste
- Lettuce (optional)
- Tomato (optional)

Instructions:

- In a bowl, combine tuna, cottage cheese, mayonnaise, celery, red onion, and dill (if using).

- Season with salt and pepper to taste.
- Spread the tuna mixture evenly on one slice of toasted bread.
- Add lettuce and tomato (optional) for extra flavor and texture.
- Place the last piece of toast on top.

Total Preparation Time: 10 minutes

Servings: one

Nutritional Information (approximate per serving):
Calories: 350
Protein: 30g
Carbohydrates: 35g
Fat: 10g

Tips:

- For a creamier texture, mash the cottage cheese slightly before mixing it with the tuna.
- For a taste of refreshment, squeeze in some lemon juice.

- You can use chopped fresh herbs like parsley or chives instead of dill.
- Substitute whole-wheat bread with whole-wheat pita bread for a different presentation.

Shrimp Scampi with Whole-Wheat Pasta and Asparagus

Ingredients:

- 1 pound shrimp peeled and deveined.
- 1 tablespoon olive oil
- 3 cloves garlic, minced.
- 1/2 cup dry white wine
- 1 cup low-sodium chicken broth
- 1/2 cup chopped cherry tomatoes.
- 1/2-pound whole-wheat pasta (penne, spaghetti, etc.)
- One bunch of asparagus, thinly sliced into small pieces.
- 1/4 cup chopped fresh parsley.
- Salt and freshly ground black pepper to taste.
- Lemon wedges (optional)

Instructions:

- Cook the whole-wheat pasta according to package instructions. Drain and set aside.
- Heat the olive oil in a big pan over medium heat while the pasta cooks.
- Once the shrimp are pink and opaque, grill them for two to three minutes on each side. Take out of the pan and place aside.
- When the garlic is aromatic, add it to the pan and simmer for 30 seconds.
- After adding the white wine, scrape away any browned pieces from the pan's bottom.
- After a minute of simmering the wine, add the cherry tomatoes and chicken broth.
- After bringing to a boil, lower heat, and simmer for five minutes.
- Add asparagus and cook for 2-3 minutes, or until tender-crisp.
- Add cooked shrimp and pasta back to the pan.
- Combine all ingredients and toss to cover with sauce.

- Season with salt and pepper to taste.
- Garnish with fresh parsley and serve with lemon wedges (optional).

Cooking Time: 15 minutes

Total Preparation Time: 20 minutes

Servings: 4

Nutritional Information (approximate per serving):
Calories: 450
Protein: 35g
Carbohydrates: 50g
Fat: 15g

Tips:

- You can use frozen shrimp, but thaw them completely before cooking.
- If you don't have white wine, you can substitute it with chicken broth or water.
- For some added spiciness, add a little sprinkle of red pepper flakes.
- To finish the dish, serve with a side salad.

High-Protein Chicken Soup with Brown Rice

Ingredients:

- 1 tablespoon olive oil
- 1 medium onion, chopped.
- 2 carrots, chopped.
- 2 celery stalks, chopped.
- 4 cloves garlic, minced.
- 1-pound boneless, skinless chicken breast, chopped
- 8 cups low-sodium chicken broth
- 1 cup brown rice, rinsed.
- 1 teaspoon dried thyme
- 1/2 teaspoon dried parsley
- Salt and black pepper to taste
- Chopped fresh herbs (optional) - chives, parsley, dill.

Instructions:

- In a big saucepan, warm up the olive oil over medium heat. Add the celery, carrots, and onion. Simmer for five minutes, or until tender.

- Add the garlic and simmer, stirring, for one more minute, or until fragrant.
- Add chicken breast, chicken broth, brown rice, thyme, and parsley. Bring to a boil, then reduce heat and simmer for 30 minutes, or until rice is cooked through and chicken is cooked to 165°F internal temperature.
- Season with salt and pepper to taste.

Cooking Time: 30 minutes

Total Preparation Time: 10 minutes

Servings: 4

Nutritional Value (per serving):
Calories: 400
Protein: 35g
Carbohydrates: 30g
Fat: 10g

Tips:

- For a thicker soup, remove 1/2 cup of cooked vegetables and rice before blending them with an immersion blender and then return the mixture to the pot.

- For this dish, you may use any leftover cooked chicken breast.

- Add other chopped vegetables like zucchini or mushrooms for additional flavor and nutrients.

Tofu and Veggie Stir-Fry with Quinoa

Ingredients:

- One 14-oz block of firm tofu that has been drained and pressed.

- 1 tablespoon cornstarch

- 2 tablespoons soy sauce (low sodium preferred)

- 1 tablespoon vegetable oil

- 1 cup assorted vegetables (broccoli florets, bell peppers, carrots), chopped.

- 1 cup cooked quinoa

- 1/2 cup low-sodium vegetable broth

- 1 tablespoon rice vinegar

- 1 teaspoon grated ginger

- 1 clove garlic, minced.
- 1/4 teaspoon sesame oil
- Salt and black pepper to taste

Instructions:

- Cut tofu into bite-sized cubes. Toss with cornstarch and soy sauce. Set aside for 10 minutes.
- On medium-high heat, heat the vegetable oil in a big skillet or wok. When golden brown, add the tofu and cook for five to seven minutes on each side. Once taken out of the pan, place aside.
- Add chopped vegetables to the pan and cook for 3-4 minutes, or until tender-crisp.
- Stir in vegetable broth, rice vinegar, ginger, garlic, and sesame oil. Bring to a simmer and cook for 1 minute.
- Add cooked tofu and quinoa back to the pan. Toss to coat with the sauce.
- Season with salt and pepper to taste.

Cooking Time: 15 minutes

Total Preparation Time: 10 minutes

Servings: 2

Nutritional Value (per serving):
Calories: 350
Protein: 20g
Carbohydrates: 40g
Fat: 15g

Tips:

- Use a non-stick pan to prevent sticking.
- If you don't have a press for tofu, you can weigh it down with a heavy object for 10-15 minutes after draining.
- You can substitute quinoa with brown rice or another whole grain.
- Feel free to add any additional veggies you choose.

Chickpea Salad Pita with Vegetables

Ingredients:

- 1 (15-oz) can chickpeas, drained and rinsed
- 1/2 cup chopped celery.
- 1/4 cup chopped red onion.
- 1/4 cup chopped cucumber.

- 1/4 cup chopped fresh parsley.
- 2 tablespoons low-fat plain yogurt
- 1 tablespoon lemon juice
- 1 tablespoon olive oil
- 1/2 teaspoon dried oregano
- Salt and freshly ground black pepper to taste
- 2 whole-wheat pitas
- Lettuce leaves
- Sliced tomato (optional)
- Chopped avocado (optional, in moderation)

Instructions:

- In a medium bowl, mash the chickpeas with a fork until slightly crumbled. You can leave some whole chickpeas for texture.
- Add the celery, red onion, cucumber, parsley, yogurt, lemon juice, olive oil, oregano, salt, and pepper. Mix well to combine.
- Warm the whole-wheat pitas in a toaster oven or microwave according to package instructions. (Optional)

- Spread the chickpea salad evenly on the warmed pitas.
- Top with lettuce leaves, sliced tomato (optional), and a sprinkle of chopped avocado (optional, in moderation).

Total Preparation Time: 15 minutes

Servings: 2

Nutritional Information (per serving):
Calories: 350 (approx.)
Protein: 15g (approx.)
Carbohydrates: 40g (approx.)
Fat: 15g (approx.)

Tips:

- For a spicier flavor, add a pinch of red pepper flakes to the chickpea salad.
- You can use any type of chopped vegetables you like in the salad.
- If you don't have fresh herbs, you can use 1 teaspoon dried parsley.

- Leftover chickpea salad can be stored in an airtight container in the refrigerator for up to 3 days.

Salmon with Quinoa Salad

Ingredients:

- 2 salmon fillets (4-6 oz each)
- 1 tablespoon olive oil
- Salt and freshly ground black pepper to taste
- 1 cup quinoa, rinsed
- 1 1/2 cups low-fat vegetable broth
- 1 cup chopped cucumber
- 1/2 cup chopped red bell pepper
- 1/4 cup chopped red onion
- 2 tablespoons chopped fresh dill or parsley
- 2 tablespoons lemon juice
- 1 tablespoon olive oil

Instructions:

- Preheat oven to 400°F (200°C).
- Pat the salmon fillets dry with paper towels. Add salt and pepper to both sides for seasoning.
- The salmon should be put on a parchment paper-lined baking sheet. Drizzle with 1 tablespoon olive oil.

- Bake for 15-20 minutes, or until cooked through and flaky.
- While the salmon is baking, cook the quinoa. In a saucepan, combine the rinsed quinoa and vegetable broth. Bring to a boil, then reduce heat, cover, and simmer for 15 minutes, or until the quinoa is cooked through and fluffy.
- In a large bowl, combine the cooked quinoa, cucumber, red bell pepper, red onion, dill (or parsley), lemon juice, and 1 tablespoon olive oil. Season with salt and pepper to taste.
- To serve, place a salmon fillet on a plate and spoon the quinoa salad alongside.

Cooking Time: 15-20 minutes for salmon, 15 minutes for quinoa

Total Preparation Time: 30-35 minutes

Servings: 2

Nutritional Information (per serving):
Calories: 450 (approx.)
Protein: 30g (approx.)

Carbohydrates: 40g (approx.)
Fat: 15g (approx.)

Tips:

- You can use any type of fresh herbs you like in the quinoa salad, such as cilantro or chives.
- If you don't have fresh lemon juice, you can use 1 tablespoon bottled lemon juice.
- Leftover quinoa salad can be stored in an airtight container in the refrigerator for up to 5 days.

Türkiye and Vegetable Wrap with Cottage Cheese

Ingredients:

- 1 whole-wheat tortilla
- 3 ounces sliced skinless turkey breast.
- 1/2 cup chopped romaine lettuce.
- 1/4 cup chopped tomato.
- 1/4 cup shredded carrots
- 2 tablespoons low-fat cottage cheese
- 1 tablespoon light mayonnaise (optional)

- Salt and pepper to taste

Instructions:

- *Prepare the vegetables:* Wash and chop the romaine lettuce, tomato, and carrots.
- *Assemble the wrap:* Spread the cottage cheese evenly on the whole-wheat tortilla. Layer the sliced turkey breast, chopped romaine lettuce, tomato, and carrots on top of the cottage cheese.
- *Seasoning (optional):* Add a pinch of salt and pepper to taste.
- *Wrap it up:* Carefully fold the bottom of the tortilla over the filling, then fold it in the sides. Roll the tortilla tightly to enclose the filling.

Total Preparation Time: 5 minutes

Servings: 1

Nutritional Information (approximate values per serving):
Calories: 300
Protein: 25g

Carbohydrates: 30g
Fat: 5g (depending on mayonnaise use)

Tips:

- For added flavor, spread a thin layer of light mayonnaise on the tortilla before adding the cottage cheese.
- You can add other vegetables to the wrap, such as sliced cucumber, bell peppers, or spinach.
- If you don't have low-fat cottage cheese, you can substitute with an equal amount of shredded low-fat cheddar cheese.
- For a vegetarian option, replace the turkey breast with sliced tofu or tempeh, marinated and cooked beforehand.
- Feel free to toast the whole-wheat tortilla in a dry skillet for a slightly crispy texture.

Dinner recipes

Baked Cod with Lemon and Herbs, Quinoa

Ingredients:

- 1 cod fillet (4-6 oz)
- 1 tablespoon olive oil
- 1/2 lemon, juiced.
- 1 teaspoon dried thyme
- 1/2 teaspoon dried parsley
- Salt and black pepper to taste
- 1 cup quinoa, rinsed.
- 1 1/2 cups low-sodium vegetable broth

Instructions:

- Preheat oven to 400°F (200°C). Line a baking sheet with parchment paper.
- Pat the cod fillet dry with paper towels. Place the cod on the prepared baking sheet.
- Drizzle the cod with olive oil, lemon juice, and sprinkle with thyme, parsley, salt, and pepper.
- In a separate pot, combine the rinsed quinoa and vegetable broth. Bring to a boil, then reduce heat, cover, and simmer for 15 minutes or until quinoa is fluffy and cooked through.

- Bake the cod for 12-15 minutes, or until the fish flakes easily with a fork.
- Fluff the cooked quinoa with a fork.

Cooking Time: 12-15 minutes for the cod, 15 minutes for the quinoa

Total Preparation Time: 25-30 minutes

Servings: 1

Nutritional Value (approximate per serving):
Calories: 400
Protein: 30g
Carbohydrates: 40g
Fat: 10g

Tips:

- You can substitute cod with other lean white fish like tilapia or haddock.
- Add other herbs like rosemary or oregano for a different flavor profile.
- Serve the cod with a side of steamed vegetables for additional nutrients.

Türkiye Breast with Brown Rice and Steamed Broccoli

Ingredients:

- 4 oz boneless, skinless turkey breast
- 1/2 teaspoon olive oil
- Salt and black pepper to taste
- 1/2 cup brown rice, rinsed.
- 1 cup low-sodium chicken broth
- 1 cup broccoli florets

Instructions:

- Preheat oven to 375°F (190°C). Lightly grease a baking dish.
- Season the turkey breast with salt and pepper. Place the turkey breast in the prepared baking dish. Drizzle with olive oil.
- In a separate pot, combine the rinsed brown rice and chicken broth. Bring to a boil, then reduce heat, cover, and simmer for 45 minutes or until rice is fluffy and cooked through.
- While the rice cooks, steam the broccoli florets for 5-7 minutes, or until tender-crisp.

- Bake the turkey breast for 20-25 minutes, or until cooked through (internal temperature reaches 165°F/74°C).
- Slice the turkey breast and serve with the cooked brown rice and steamed broccoli.

Cooking Time: 20-25 minutes for the turkey breast, 45 minutes for the brown rice, 5-7 minutes for the broccoli

Total Preparation Time: 1 hour (depending on rice cooking time)

Servings: 1

Nutritional Value (approximate per serving):
Calories: 450
Protein: 40g
Carbohydrates: 45g
Fat: 5g

Tips:

- You can marinate the turkey breast in low-fat yogurt with herbs for added flavor before baking.

- Substitute brown rice with quinoa or another whole grain for a different texture.
- Drizzle the steamed broccoli with a touch of lemon juice or low-fat vinaigrette dressing.

Shrimp and Vegetable Curry with Quinoa

Ingredients:

- 1 tablespoon olive oil
- 1 medium onion, chopped
- 2 cloves garlic, minced
- 1 tablespoon curry powder
- 1 teaspoon ground ginger
- 1/2 teaspoon turmeric
- 1 (14.5 oz) can diced tomatoes, undrained
- 1 (13.5 oz) can light coconut milk
- 1 cup vegetable broth
- 1 cup quinoa, rinsed
- 1 pound shrimp, peeled and deveined (thawed if frozen)
- 1 cup assorted vegetables (broccoli florets, bell pepper strips, sugar snap peas)
- 1 tablespoon chopped fresh cilantro (optional)
- Cooked brown rice (optional, for serving)
- Lime wedges (for serving)

Instructions:

- In a big saucepan or Dutch oven, warm up the olive oil over medium heat. Add the onion and simmer for approximately 5 minutes, or until softened. Add the turmeric, ginger, garlic, and curry powder and stir. Cook, stirring regularly, for a further minute.

- Add the veggie broth, coconut milk, and chopped tomatoes. After bringing to a boil, lower the heat and simmer. Cook with a cover on for ten minutes.

- Stir in rinsed quinoa and return to a simmer. Cook according to package directions, about 15 minutes, or until quinoa is fluffy and cooked through.

- In the last 5 minutes of cooking, add shrimp and vegetables. Stir gently until shrimp are pink and opaque, and vegetables are tender-crisp.

- Remove from heat and stir in chopped cilantro (if using).

Cooking Time: 25 minutes (excluding quinoa cooking time)

Total Preparation Time: 35 minutes (including quinoa cooking time)

Servings: 4

Nutritional Information (per serving):
Calories: 450
Protein: 30g
Carbohydrates: 50g
Fat: 15g

Tips:

- For a thicker curry, use less vegetable broth or simmer for a few minutes longer after adding the shrimp and vegetables.

- Substitute other vegetables like carrots, zucchini, or green beans.

- Serve over cooked brown rice for a more filling meal.

- Adjust the curry powder amount to your desired spice level.

Tofu Veggie Burgers on Whole-Wheat Buns with Sweet Potato Fries

Ingredients:

For the Tofu Burgers:

- One 14-oz block of firm tofu that has been drained and pressed.
- 1 cup cooked brown rice.
- 1/2 cup chopped red onion.
- 1/2 cup chopped bell pepper (any color)
- 1/4 cup chopped fresh parsley.
- 2 cloves garlic, minced.
- 1 tablespoon soy sauce (low sodium preferred)
- 1 tablespoon olive oil
- 1/2 teaspoon ground cumin
- 1/4 teaspoon smoked paprika.
- 1/4 teaspoon black pepper
- 1/4 cup panko breadcrumbs (whole-wheat preferred)

For the Sweet Potato Fries:

- 1 large, sweet potato, peeled and cut into wedges
- 1 tablespoon olive oil
- 1/2 teaspoon dried thyme
- 1/4 teaspoon garlic powder
- Pinch of cayenne pepper (optional)
- Salt and freshly ground black pepper to taste.

For Serving:

- 2 whole-wheat hamburger buns
- Lettuce leaves, sliced tomato, sliced red onion (optional)
- Your favorite low-fat condiments (ketchup, mustard, etc.)

Instructions:

- ***Prepare the Tofu Burgers:*** Preheat oven to 400°F (200°C). Wrap the drained tofu in a clean kitchen towel and press out any excess moisture. Put the tofu in a big basin and crumble it.
- Add cooked brown rice, chopped vegetables (red onion, bell pepper, parsley), minced

garlic, soy sauce, olive oil, spices (cumin, paprika, black pepper), and panko breadcrumbs to the bowl with the tofu. Mix well to combine.

- Form the mixture into two equal patties. Arrange the patties onto a parchment paper-lined baking sheet. Bake for 20 minutes, then flip and bake for an additional 10-15 minutes, or until golden brown and firm to the touch.

- *Prepare the Sweet Potato Fries:* While the burgers bake, preheat oven to 425°F (220°C). Toss sweet potato wedges with olive oil, dried thyme, garlic powder, cayenne pepper (optional), salt, and black pepper. Arrange the fries in a single layer on a baking pan.

- Bake for 20-25 minutes, or until tender and slightly crispy, flipping halfway through cooking.

Cooking Time:

Tofu Burgers: 30-35 minutes

Sweet Potato Fries: 20-25 minutes

Total Preparation Time: 45-50 minutes

Serving Size: 2 burgers with sweet potato fries

Nutritional Information (approximate per serving):
Calories: 500-600
Protein: 20-25 grams
Carbohydrates: 60-70 grams
Fat: 20-25 grams (depending on oil used)

Tips:

- To press the tofu, place it on a cutting board, top it with another cutting board, and weigh it down with a heavy object (like a can of beans) for 30 minutes.
- You can add other chopped vegetables to the burger mixture, such as carrots, mushrooms, or zucchini.
- For a spicier burger, add a pinch of red pepper flakes to the mixture.
- Serve the burgers on lettuce wraps instead of buns for a lower-carb option.

- Dip the sweet potato fries in your favorite low-fat yogurt or hummus sauce for added protein and flavor.

Chicken and Vegetable Kabobs with Brown Rice

Ingredients:

- one pound of skin-and bone-free chicken breasts, cubed into 1-inch pieces.
- One bell pepper, diced into 1-inch squares (orange, yellow, or red).
- One medium red onion, thinly sliced into 1-inch pieces.
- 1 zucchini, cut into 1-inch pieces.
- 1 tablespoon olive oil
- 1 tablespoon lemon juice
- 1 teaspoon dried oregano
- 1/2 teaspoon garlic powder
- Salt and black pepper to taste
- 1 cup cooked brown rice (per serving)

- Wooden skewers (to avoid scorching, immerse them in water for at least half an hour)

Instructions:

- *Prep (10 minutes):* In a large bowl, combine olive oil, lemon juice, oregano, garlic powder, salt, and pepper. To ensure uniform coating, add the chicken pieces and mix. Marinate for at least 30 minutes (or up to 2 hours) in the refrigerator.

- *Assemble Kabobs (5 minutes):* Thread chicken cubes, bell pepper squares, onion wedges, and zucchini pieces alternately onto soaked wooden skewers.

- *Cooking (15-20 minutes):* Preheat grill to medium-high heat. Grill kabobs for 15-20 minutes, turning occasionally, until chicken is cooked through and vegetables are tender-crisp. You can also bake them in a preheated oven at 400°F (200°C) for 20-25 minutes, flipping halfway through.

- ***Serve (2 minutes):*** Plate cooked kabobs with a side of brown rice.

Total Preparation Time: 27-47 minutes (depending on marinating time and cooking method)

Servings: 4

Nutritional Information (per serving with brown rice):
Calories: Around 400 (depending on the specific ingredients used)
Protein: Around 30 grams
Carbohydrates: Around 40 grams (including fiber)
Fat: Around 10 grams

Tips:

- Marinate the chicken for a longer time for deeper flavor.
- For a vegetarian option, substitute tofu cubes for the chicken. Marinate the tofu in the same way.

- Play around with different vegetables like cherry tomatoes, mushrooms, or broccoli florets.
- Serve with a low-fat yogurt sauce or a light vinaigrette dressing for dipping.
- You may keep leftover kabobs in the fridge for up to three days if you put them in an airtight container. Warm up the food slowly in the oven or on the burner.

Lentil Shepherd's Pie with Protein-Fortified Mashed Potatoes

Ingredients:

For the Lentil Filling:

- 1 tablespoon olive oil
- 1 medium onion, chopped.
- 2 carrots, chopped.
- 2 celery stalks, chopped.
- 2 cloves garlic, minced.
- 1 cup brown lentils, rinsed.
- 4 cups low-fat vegetable broth
- 1 (14.5 oz) can diced tomatoes, undrained

- 1 teaspoon dried thyme
- 1/2 teaspoon dried rosemary
- Salt and freshly ground black pepper to taste.

For the Protein-Fortified Mashed Potatoes:

- 2 pounds russet potatoes, peeled and cubed
- 1 cup low-fat milk
- 1/4 cup low-fat cottage cheese
- 1 scoop protein powder (unflavored or savory, approved by your doctor)
- 1 tablespoon butter
- Salt and freshly ground black pepper to taste.

Instructions:

- ***Get the lentil filling ready:*** In a big saucepan or Dutch oven, warm up the olive oil over medium heat. Add the celery, carrots, and onion. Sauté until softened, about 5 to 7 minutes.
- Cook the garlic for one more minute, or until aromatic.

- Add the diced tomatoes, vegetable broth, thyme, and rosemary once the lentils have been rinsed. To taste, add salt and pepper for seasoning.
- Once the lentils are cooked, simmer for 20 to 25 minutes on low heat after bringing them to a boil.

Prepare the Protein-Fortified Mashed Potatoes:

- While the lentils cook, place cubed potatoes in a large pot and cover with water. After bringing to a boil, lower the heat, and simmer until the food is fork-tender, 15 to 20 minutes.
- After draining, add the potatoes back to the saucepan. Use a hand mixer or potato masher to mash.
- In a separate bowl, whisk together low-fat milk, cottage cheese, protein powder, and butter. Season with salt and pepper to taste.
- Gradually add the milk mixture to the mashed potatoes, mixing until smooth and creamy.

Assemble the Shepherd's Pie:

- Preheat oven to 375°F (190°C). Grease a 9x13 inch baking dish.
- Filling for lentils should be spooned into the baking dish.
- Top with the protein-fortified mashed potatoes, spreading evenly.
- Bake for 20-25 minutes, or until the top is golden brown and bubbly.

Cooking Time: 40-45 minutes (20-25 minutes for lentil filling, 20-25 minutes for baking)

Total Preparation Time: 1 hour

Servings: 6

Nutritional Information (per serving):
Calories: Approximately 450-500 (may vary depending on protein powder)
Protein: 30-35 grams (including protein powder)
Carbohydrates: 50-55 grams
Fat: 10-15 grams

Tips:

- You can add other vegetables to the lentil filling, such as chopped mushrooms, green peppers, or frozen peas.
- If you don't have protein powder, you can increase the amount of cottage cheese in the mashed potatoes.
- You may keep leftovers in the fridge for up to three days if you put them in an airtight container.

Baked Salmon with Roasted Brussels Sprouts and Quinoa

Ingredients:

- 1 salmon fillet (6 oz)
- 1 tablespoon olive oil
- 1/2 teaspoon dried dill
- Salt and pepper to taste
- 1 pound Brussels sprouts, trimmed and halved
- 1 cup quinoa, rinsed.
- 1 1/2 cups low-sodium vegetable broth
- 1/2 cup chopped red onion

Instructions:

- Preheat oven to 400°F (200°C). Line a baking sheet with parchment paper.
- In a small bowl, combine olive oil and dill. Season salmon fillet with salt and pepper. Brush the salmon with the olive oil mixture.
- Toss Brussels sprouts with red onion and a drizzle of olive oil. Season with salt and pepper. Spread the Brussels sprouts on one half of the prepared baking sheet.
- Transfer the salmon to the opposite side of the baking sheet.
- In a separate pot, combine quinoa and vegetable broth. Bring to a boil, then reduce heat, cover, and simmer for 15 minutes, or until quinoa is cooked and fluffy.
- Bake the salmon and Brussels sprouts for 15-20 minutes, or until the salmon is cooked through and the Brussels sprouts are tender-crisp.
- Fluff the quinoa with a fork.

Cooking Time: 35 minutes (including quinoa cooking)

Total Preparation Time: 45 minutes

Servings: 2

Nutritional Information (per serving):
Calories: 450
Protein: 35g
Carbohydrates: 40g
Fat: 15g

Tips:

- You can substitute other herbs like parsley or lemon pepper seasoning for dill.
- Add a squeeze of fresh lemon juice to the salmon before baking for extra flavor.
- For a vegetarian option, replace the salmon with a block of firm tofu, marinated in your favorite low-sodium sauce, and bake alongside the Brussels sprouts.

Flank Steak Fajitas with Whole-Wheat Tortillas

Ingredients:

- 1 pound flank steak thinly sliced.

- 1 tablespoon olive oil

- 1 teaspoon chili powder

- 1/2 teaspoon cumin

- 1/4 teaspoon smoked paprika.

- 1/4 teaspoon garlic powder

- Salt and pepper to taste

- One sliced bell pepper, either red, yellow, or orange

- 1 onion, sliced.

- 4 whole-wheat tortillas

- Optional toppings: chopped tomatoes, shredded lettuce, low-fat cheese, salsa, guacamole

Instructions:

- In a large bowl, combine the flank steak with olive oil, chili powder, cumin, smoked paprika, garlic powder, salt, and pepper. Toss to coat evenly.

- Heat a large skillet over medium-high heat. Add the marinated steak and cook for 3-4 minutes per side, or until desired doneness. Take out of the pan and place it aside.

- In the same skillet, add the bell pepper and onion. Sauté for 5-7 minutes, or until softened and slightly browned.
- The whole-wheat tortillas should be warmed per the directions on the package.
- To assemble the fajitas, place some sliced steak and vegetables on a tortilla. Add your desired toppings (optional).

Cooking Time: 15 minutes

Total Preparation Time: 20 minutes

Servings: 4

Nutritional Information (per serving without toppings):
Calories: 350
Protein: 30g
Carbohydrates: 30g
Fat: 10g

Tips:

- Marinate the flank steak for at least 30 minutes for extra flavor.
- You can use a grill pan or outdoor grill to cook the steak for a smoky flavor.
- Add other vegetables like sliced zucchini or mushrooms to the fajitas.
- Serve with a low-fat yogurt-based dipping sauce instead of sour cream.

Shrimp and Asparagus Stir-Fry with Brown Rice

Ingredients:

- 1 pound shrimp, peeled and deveined (thawed if frozen)
- 1 pound asparagus, trimmed and cut into bite-sized pieces.
- 1 tablespoon olive oil
- 2 cloves garlic, minced.
- 1 teaspoon grated ginger
- 1/4 cup low-sodium soy sauce
- 1 tablespoon rice vinegar
- 1 tablespoon cornstarch

- 2 cups cooked brown rice
- Salt and freshly ground black pepper to taste
- Chopped green onions (optional, for garnish)

Instructions:

- ***Prep (5 minutes):*** Wash and chop asparagus. Mince garlic and ginger. Prepare cooked brown rice according to package instructions (if not already cooked).
- ***Marinate Shrimp (10 minutes):*** In a medium bowl, combine cornstarch, 1 tablespoon soy sauce, and 1 tablespoon rice vinegar. Add shrimp and toss to coat. Marinate for 10 minutes.
- ***Stir-Fry (10-12 minutes):*** Heat olive oil in a large wok or skillet over medium-high heat. Cook for 30 seconds or until aromatic after adding the ginger and garlic.
- ***Add Shrimp (5 minutes):*** Add the shrimp and cook for 2-3 minutes per side, or until pink and opaque. Take the shrimp out of the pan and place it aside.

- *Cook Asparagus (3-5 minutes):* Add the asparagus to the pan and stir-fry for 3-5 minutes, or until tender-crisp.
- *Sauce and Combine (2-3 minutes):* In a small bowl, whisk together remaining soy sauce, rice vinegar, and a splash of water to create a thin sauce. Transfer the sauce to the pan containing the asparagus. Bring to a simmer and cook for 1 minute.
- *Finish and Serve:* Add cooked shrimp back to the pan and toss to combine with the sauce and asparagus. Season with salt and pepper to taste. Serve immediately over cooked brown rice. Garnish with chopped green onions (optional).

Total Preparation Time: 25 minutes

Cooking Time: 15-17 minutes

Servings: 4

Nutritional Information (per serving): (approximate values)
Calories: 450
Protein: 35g

Carbohydrates: 40g
Fat: 15g

Tips:

- You can substitute other vegetables for asparagus, such as broccoli, bell peppers, or snow peas.
- Add a splash of low-sodium chicken broth to the sauce if you prefer a richer flavor.
- Serve with a side of low-fat steamed edamame for additional protein and fiber.
- Use a non-stick pan for easier cleaning.

Chicken Breast with Quinoa and Roasted Vegetables

Ingredients:

- 1 boneless, skinless chicken breast (around 150g)
- 1 cup quinoa, rinsed.
- 1.5 cups low-sodium chicken broth
- 1 tablespoon olive oil
- 1 red bell pepper, sliced.
- 1 yellow bell pepper, sliced.

- 1 medium zucchini, sliced.

- 1/2 red onion, sliced.

- 1/2 teaspoon dried oregano

- 1/4 teaspoon dried thyme

- Salt and black pepper to taste

- Fresh parsley (optional, for garnish)

Instructions:

- Preheat oven to 400°F (200°C). Line a baking sheet with parchment paper.

- *Prepare the quinoa:* In a saucepan, combine rinsed quinoa with chicken broth. Bring to a boil, then reduce heat, cover, and simmer for 15 minutes or until cooked through and fluffy. Set it aside.

- *Marinate the chicken:* In a small bowl, combine olive oil, oregano, thyme, salt, and pepper. Place the chicken breast in the bowl and coat it evenly with the marinade. Let it sit for 10 minutes while preparing the vegetables.

- *Roast the vegetables:* Toss bell pepper slices, zucchini slices, and red onion slices with a drizzle of olive oil and a pinch of salt and pepper. On the baking sheet that has been prepared, distribute the veggies equally.

- *Bake the chicken and vegetables:* Place the marinated chicken breast on top of the vegetables on the baking sheet. Bake for 20-25 minutes, or until the chicken is cooked through (internal temperature reaches 165°F/74°C) and the vegetables are tender-crisp.

- *Assemble and serve:* Fluff the cooked quinoa with a fork. Divide the quinoa among plates. Top with a roasted chicken breast and roasted vegetables. Garnish with fresh parsley (optional).

Cooking Time: 20-25 minutes

Total Preparation Time: 40 minutes

Serving Size: 1 person

Nutritional Information (approximate per serving):
Calories: 400-450

Protein: 40-45g
Carbohydrates: 40-45g (including fiber)
Fat: 10-15g

Tips:

- You can use other vegetables in this recipe, such as broccoli florets, asparagus spears, or cherry tomatoes. Simply adjust the roasting time based on the thickness of the vegetables.
- You may keep leftovers in the fridge for up to three days if you put them in an airtight container. Prior to serving, reheat gently in the oven or microwave.
- For added flavor, you can marinate the chicken in your favorite spices, such as paprika, cumin, or chili powder.
- Feel free to adjust the amount of herbs and spices to your preference.

Snacks recipes

Hard-boiled Eggs with Cottage Cheese

Ingredients:

- Two large eggs
- ½ cup low-fat cottage cheese
- Salt and pepper to taste (optional)
- Fresh herbs (optional, for garnish)

Instructions:

- Put the eggs in a saucepan in a single layer. Place a lid on the freezing water and heat it to a boiling point.
- Once boiling, remove the pan from the heat, cover, and let sit for 12 minutes for a medium-cooked yolk. For a harder yolk, cook for 15 minutes.
- Drain the hot water and immediately run icy water over the eggs to stop the cooking process. Run icy water over the eggs to peel them.
- Divide cottage cheese onto two plates. Slice the eggs in half and arrange them on top of the cottage cheese. Season with salt and pepper (optional).

- Garnish with fresh herbs like chives or parsley (optional).

Cooking Time: 12-15 minutes (after reaching a boil)

Total Preparation Time: 15-20 minutes

Serving Size: 1 person

Nutritional Information (approximate):
Calories: 230
Protein: 20g
Carbohydrates: 5g
Fat: 12g

Tips:

- For easier peeling, place the eggs in a bowl of cold water after cooking and let them sit for a few minutes before peeling.
- You can add a sprinkle of paprika or other spices for additional flavor.
- Hard-boiled eggs can be made ahead of time and stored in the refrigerator for up to a week.

Edamame Pods with a Sprinkle of Chili Flakes

Ingredients:

- 1 cup frozen edamame pods, in the shell
- ½ teaspoon olive oil
- Pinch of chili flakes (adjust to your spice preference)
- Sea salt to taste

Instructions:

- If using frozen edamame, thaw according to package instructions. You can thaw them in the microwave, following the power and time recommendations, or by placing them in a colander and running cold water over them for a few minutes.
- The olive oil should be warmed in a pan over medium heat. Add the edamame pods and chili flakes.
- Sauté for 2-3 minutes, stirring occasionally, until the edamame pods are heated through and slightly blistered.

- Sprinkle with sea salt to taste.

Cooking Time: 2-3 minutes

Total Preparation Time: 5-10 minutes

Serving Size: 1 person

Nutritional Information (approximate):
Calories: 120
Protein: 12g
Carbohydrates: 10g
Fat: 5g

Tips:

- You can use fresh edamame pods if available, but frozen edamame is a convenient option.
- Adapt the quantity of chili flakes to your desired level of spiciness.
- For a smoky flavor, sprinkle the edamame with smoked paprika instead of chili flakes.

Greek Yogurt with Protein Powder and Berries.

Ingredients:

- 1 cup low-fat Greek yogurt

- 1 scoop protein powder (approved by your doctor)
- ½ cup fresh or frozen berries
- 1 tablespoon chopped nuts and/or seeds (optional)
- Drizzle of honey or maple syrup (optional)

Instructions:

- In a bowl, combine the Greek yogurt and protein powder. Stir until well combined and smooth.
- Fold in the berries.
- Top with chopped nuts and/or seeds (optional).
- Drizzle with honey or maple syrup for additional sweetness (optional).

Total Preparation Time: 5 minutes

Serving Size: 1 person

Nutritional Information (approximate, will vary depending on protein powder and optional ingredients):
Calories: 250-300

Protein: 20-25g
Carbohydrates: 20-30g
Fat: 5-10g

Tips:

- Choose a protein powder that is flavored or unflavored depending on your preference. Make sure it's approved by your doctor for use with pancreatitis.

- You can use a variety of berries, such as blueberries, strawberries, raspberries, or blackberries.

- For a thicker consistency, use thicker Greek yogurt options.

- This recipe is easily customizable. You can add other toppings like chopped fruit, granola, or a sprinkle of cinnamon.

Trail Mix with Whole-Wheat Cereal, Dried Cranberries, and Almonds

Ingredients:

- 2 cups whole-wheat cereal (flakes, puffs, or squares)

- 1 cup dried cranberries (unsweetened or lightly sweetened)
- ½ cup almonds (raw or roasted, unsalted)

Instructions:

- In a large bowl, combine the whole-wheat cereal, dried cranberries, and almonds.
- For the ingredients to be distributed evenly, thoroughly mix.

Total Preparation Time: 5 minutes

Serving Size: ½ cup (can be adjusted based on calorie needs)

Nutritional Information (approximate per ½ cup serving):
Calories: 200
Protein: 5 grams
Carbohydrates: 30 grams
Fat: 5 grams
Fiber: 3 grams

Tips:

- For a sweeter mix, add a handful of raisins or chopped dried dates.

- Substitute other nuts like cashews or pistachios for almonds, keeping the portion size similar.

- For a more kid-friendly version, use chopped dried apricots or mango instead of cranberries.

- Store the trail mix in an airtight container at room temperature for up to a week.

Sliced Türkiye Breast with Cucumber Slices

Ingredients:

- 4 ounces sliced turkey breast (deli sliced or cooked at home)

- 1 medium cucumber, sliced.

Instructions:

- Wash the cucumber and slice it into rounds or sticks.

- Arrange the turkey slices on a plate and add the cucumber slices alongside.

Total Preparation Time: 2 minutes

Serving Size: 4 ounces sliced turkey breast and a handful of cucumber slices

Nutritional Information (approximate per serving):
Calories: 120
Protein: 25 grams
Carbohydrates: 0 grams
Fat: 3 grams
Fiber: 0 grams

Tips:

- For a touch of flavor, add a sprinkle of dried herbs like oregano or thyme to the turkey slices.
- Serve with a dollop of low-fat mustard or a light vinaigrette dressing for dipping the cucumber slices.
- If using deli sliced turkey, choose options labeled "low sodium" or "no added sodium" for better heart health.

High-Protein Smoothie

Ingredients:

- 1 cup low-fat milk (dairy or plant-based)
- ½ cup low-fat Greek yogurt
- 1 scoop protein powder (approved by your doctor)
- ½ cup frozen spinach
- ½ cup frozen berries (blueberries, raspberries, strawberries)
- ¼ cup water (optional, adjust for desired consistency)

Instructions:

- Add all ingredients to a blender.
- Blend until smooth and creamy. If the mixture is too thick, add a little water for desired consistency.
- Pour into a glass and enjoy!

Total Preparation Time: 5 minutes

Serving Size: 1

Nutritional Information (approximate per serving):
Calories: 300
Protein: 30 grams

Carbohydrates: 30 grams
Fat: 5 grams
Fiber: 4 grams

Tips:

- For a sweeter smoothie, add a ripe banana or a squeeze of honey.
- Substitute the berries with other frozen fruits like mango or pineapple.
- Use nut butter (almond butter or peanut butter) for a thicker and more flavorful smoothie, but be mindful of portion size due to added calories and fat.
- Add a handful of chopped kale or other leafy greens for an extra nutrient boost.

Cottage Cheese with Sliced Bell Peppers

Ingredients:

- 1 cup low-fat cottage cheese
- One sliced bell pepper (either red, yellow, orange, or green)
- Freshly ground black pepper (to taste)

- Optional: Chopped fresh herbs (parsley, chives, dill)

Instructions:

- In a bowl, combine cottage cheese and sliced bell peppers.
- Season with black pepper to taste.
- (Optional) Stir in chopped fresh herbs for additional flavor.

Total Preparation Time: 5 minutes

Serving Size: 1

Nutritional Information (approximate per serving):
Calories: 160
Protein: 14g
Carbohydrates: 10g
Fat: 5g

Tips:

- Use a variety of colorful bell peppers for added visual appeal and a range of vitamins.

- For a creamier texture, mash some of the cottage cheese before combining it with the peppers.
- Drizzle with a splash of olive oil or balsamic vinegar for extra flavor.

Baked Chicken Breast Strips with Low-Fat Yogurt Dip

Ingredients:

- 1 boneless, skinless chicken breast half
- 1 tablespoon olive oil
- 1/2 teaspoon dried oregano
- 1/4 teaspoon garlic powder
- Salt and black pepper (to taste)

For the Dip:

- 1/2 cup low-fat plain Greek yogurt
- 1 tablespoon chopped fresh dill (or other herbs like chives)
- 1/4 teaspoon lemon juice
- Salt and black pepper (to taste)

Instructions:

- Preheat oven to 400°F (200°C). Line a baking sheet with parchment paper.
- Cut the chicken breast into thin strips.
- Olive oil, oregano, garlic powder, salt, and pepper should all be combined in a basin. Toss the chicken strips in the marinade to coat evenly.
- Arrange the chicken strips on the prepared baking sheet.
- Bake for 15 to 20 minutes, or until well cooked and browned.
- While the chicken bakes, prepare the dip: In a small bowl, combine yogurt, dill, lemon juice, salt, and pepper. Mix well.
- Let the chicken cool slightly before serving with the yogurt dip.

Cooking Time: 15-20 minutes

Total Preparation Time: 25 minutes

Serving Size: 1

Nutritional Information (approximate per serving - with yogurt dip):
Calories: 250

Protein: 35g	
Carbohydrates: 5g	
Fat: 8g	

Tips:

- Marinate the chicken for at least 30 minutes for extra flavor.
- You can adjust the spices in the marinade to your liking (e.g., paprika, cumin).
- Serve the chicken strips with a side of steamed vegetables for a complete meal.
- Use low-fat yogurt with no added sugar for the dip.

Air-Popped Popcorn with Nutritional Yeast

Ingredients:

- 1/4 cup popcorn kernels
- 1 tablespoon olive oil (optional)
- 1 tablespoon nutritional yeast

Instructions:

- Heat an air popper according to the manufacturer's instructions.

- Add the popcorn kernels and pop according to the air popper's instructions.
- (Optional) While the popcorn is popping, heat the olive oil in a small pan over low heat.
- When the popcorn is all popped, move it into a big bowl.
- Sprinkle the nutritional yeast over the popcorn.
- (Optional) Drizzle with the warmed olive oil, if using, to help the nutritional yeast adhere.
- Toss to coat the popcorn evenly.

Cooking Time: Varies depending on air popper (around 5 minutes)

Total Preparation Time: 10 minutes

Serving Size: 1-2

Nutritional Information (approximate per serving):
Calories: 120
Protein: 3g

Carbohydrates: 20g
Fat: 5g

Tips:

- Popcorn kernels are a whole grain, providing some fiber.
- Nutritional yeast is a deactivated yeast that adds a cheesy flavor and a slight protein boost.
- You can adjust the amount of nutritional yeast to your taste preference.
- Experiment with other seasonings on your popcorn, such as garlic powder or smoked paprika.

Roasted Chickpeas with Spices

Ingredients:

- 1 (15-ounce) can chickpeas, drained and rinsed
- 1 tablespoon olive oil
- 1/2 teaspoon ground cumin
- 1/2 teaspoon smoked paprika
- 1/4 teaspoon garlic powder

- 1/4 teaspoon chili powder (optional, for heat)
- Salt and freshly ground black pepper, to taste.

Instructions:

- Preheat oven to 400°F (200°C). Line a baking sheet with parchment paper.
- Pat the chickpeas dry with a clean kitchen towel to remove any excess moisture. This ensures they crisp up nicely during roasting.
- In a large bowl, toss the chickpeas with olive oil, cumin, paprika, garlic powder, chili powder (if using), salt, and pepper. Make sure all the chickpeas are evenly coated with the spice mixture.
- Spread the chickpeas on the prepared baking sheet in a single layer. Avoid overcrowding the pan, as this will prevent them from crisping evenly.
- Roast for 20-25 minutes, or until the chickpeas are golden brown and slightly

crispy. Shake the pan occasionally to achieve uniform roasting.

- Remove from the oven and allow to cool slightly before serving.

Cooking Time: 20-25 minutes

Total Preparation Time: 30 minutes (including preheating)

Servings: 4-6 (as a snack)

Nutritional Value (per serving):
Calories: 190
Fat: 6g
Saturated Fat: 1g
Cholesterol: 0mg
Sodium: 130mg (depending on added salt)
Carbohydrates: 21g
Fiber: 6g
Protein: 8g

Tips:

- For extra flavor, add a sprinkle of cayenne pepper or a squeeze of fresh lemon juice before serving.

- You can experiment with different spice combinations. Try a blend of curry powder, coriander, and turmeric for an Indian-inspired twist.

- Roasted chickpeas can be stored in an airtight container at room temperature for up to 5 days. They make a healthy and portable snack option.

- If you do not have parchment paper, you can lightly grease the baking sheet with olive oil instead.

- To evaluate for doneness, remove a few chickpeas from the oven after 20 minutes. If they are still soft, continue roasting for a few more minutes. Be careful not to overcook them, as they can become dry and hard.

Dessert recipes

Baked Apples with Cinnamon and Protein Powder

Ingredients:

- 2 large apples (such as Granny Smith, Honeycrisp)
- 1/4 cup water
- 1/2 teaspoon ground cinnamon
- 1/4 teaspoon ground nutmeg (optional)
- 1-2 tablespoons protein powder (approved by your doctor)
- 1 tablespoon honey

Instructions:

- Preheat oven to 375°F (190°C). Lightly grease a baking dish.
- Core the apples, leaving the bottom intact. You may use either an apple corner or a little knife.
- In a small bowl, combine water, cinnamon, and nutmeg (if using).
- Place apples in the prepared baking dish. Pour the water mixture into the bottom of the dish.
- Sprinkle each apple with half the protein powder. Drizzle with honey.

- Bake for 30-35 minutes, or until apples are tender but not mushy. You can test with a fork by inserting it into the thickest part of the apple.

- Let cool slightly before serving.

Cooking Time: 30-35 minutes

Total Preparation Time: 10-15 minutes

Servings: 2

Nutritional Information (per serving):
Calories: Around 180 (depending on the protein powder and apple size)
Protein: Around 10-15 grams (depending on the protein powder)
Carbohydrates: Around 30 grams
Fat: Around 1 gram

Tips:

- For a vegan option, use a plant-based protein powder and vegan honey substitute.

- You can stuff the apples with other healthy ingredients like chopped nuts, raisins, or dried cranberries.

- Serve the baked apples with a dollop of low-fat yogurt or whipped cream for extra protein and creaminess.

High-Protein Yogurt Parfait

Ingredients:

- 1 cup low-fat Greek yogurt
- 1/2 cup sliced banana.
- 1/4 cup berries (fresh or frozen)
- 1-2 tablespoons protein powder (approved by your doctor)
- 1 tablespoon chopped nuts (almonds, walnuts, pistachios) (optional)
- 1 tablespoon granola (optional)
- A drizzle of honey (optional)

Instructions:

- In a small bowl or parfait glass, layer half of the Greek yogurt.
- Top with half of the sliced banana and half of the berries.
- Sprinkle half of the protein powder.
- Repeat layers with remaining yogurt, banana, berries, protein powder, and nuts (if using).

- Drizzle with honey (if using) and sprinkle with granola (if using) for added texture.

Total Preparation Time: 5 minutes

Servings: 1

Nutritional Information (per serving):
Calories: Around 250 (depending on the protein powder, nuts, and granola)
Protein: Around 20-25 grams (depending on the protein powder)
Carbohydrates: Around 30-40 grams
Fat: Around 5-10 grams (depending on the nuts and granola)

Tips:

- You can use different types of yogurt like vanilla or flavored Greek yogurt for a change in taste.
- Experiment with different fruits and nuts to create your own flavor combinations.
- If using frozen berries, you can thaw them slightly before layering in the parfait.

- Prepare the parfait ahead of time and store it in the refrigerator for a grab-and-go breakfast or snack.

Frozen Greek Yogurt with Berries and Protein Powder

Ingredients:

- 1 cup low-fat Greek yogurt
- 1/2 scoop protein powder (approved by your doctor)
- 1/2 cup frozen berries (blueberries, raspberries, strawberries)
- 1 tablespoon honey (optional)

Instructions:

- (Prep Time: 5 minutes) Combine the Greek yogurt, protein powder, and frozen berries in a blender.
- (Blending Time: 1-2 minutes) Blend until smooth and creamy. You may need to stop and scrape down the sides a couple of times for even blending.

- (Freezing Time: 2-3 hours or overnight) Pour the mixture into a freezer-safe container. Freeze for at least 2-3 hours, or overnight for a firmer consistency.

Total Preparation Time: 5 minutes + freezing time

Serving Size: 1

Nutritional Information (approximate values per serving):
Calories: 200-250 (depending on protein powder and yogurt)
Protein: 20-25 grams (depending on protein powder)
Carbohydrates: 20-30 grams (depending on fruit and yogurt)
Fat: 5-10 grams (depending on yogurt)

Tips:

- Use a rippled Greek yogurt for added texture.

- If the mixture seems too thick after freezing, let it sit at room temperature for a few minutes to soften slightly before scooping.
- For a more intense berry flavor, blend in a few tablespoons of fresh or frozen berries with the yogurt and protein powder.
- Top your frozen yogurt with a sprinkle of chopped nuts, granola, or a drizzle of honey for extra flavor and crunch.

Chia Seed Pudding with Protein

Ingredients:

- 1/3 cup chia seeds
- 1 cup low-fat milk (dairy or plant-based)
- 1/2 scoop protein powder (approved by your doctor)
- 1/4 teaspoon vanilla extract (optional)
- 1/4 cup sliced fresh fruit (berries, banana, mango)
- 1 tablespoon chopped nuts or seeds (almonds, walnuts, chia seeds) (optional)

Instructions:

- (Prep Time: 5 minutes) In a bowl or jar, whisk together the chia seeds, milk, protein powder, and vanilla extract (if using).
- (Soaking Time: Overnight) Cover and refrigerate for at least 8 hours, or overnight, to allow the chia seeds to absorb the liquid and thicken.
- (Serving Time: 2 minutes) Before serving, stir in the sliced fruit and chopped nuts or seeds (if using).

Total Preparation Time: 5 minutes + soaking time

Serving Size: 1

Nutritional Information (approximate values per serving):
Calories: 250-300 (depending on milk, protein powder, and toppings)
Protein: 15-20 grams (depending on protein powder)
Carbohydrates: 30-40 grams (depending on milk and fruit)

Fat: 5-10 grams (depending on milk and toppings)

Tips:

- Use several types of milk (almond, coconut) and protein powder flavors to create variety.
- For a thicker pudding, use a 2:1 ratio of chia seeds to milk.
- To add additional sweetness, sprinkle with honey or maple syrup.
- Layer the chia pudding with fruit compote or yogurt parfaits for a more layered dessert.
- You can prepare a large batch of chia pudding in advance and store it in the refrigerator for up to 4 days.

High-Protein Mug Cake

Ingredients:

- 1/4 cup whole wheat flour
- 1 scoop protein powder (approved by your doctor)
- 1/4 teaspoon baking powder
- 1/8 teaspoon salt

- 1/4 cup unsweetened almond milk (or low-fat milk)
- 1 tablespoon mashed banana (or applesauce)
- 1 tablespoon honey (or maple syrup)
- 1 teaspoon of heated coconut oil (or unsalted butter).
- Optional: 1/4 cup chopped nuts or berries

Instructions:

- In a microwave-safe mug, whisk together the dry ingredients: flour, protein powder, baking powder, and salt.
- In a separate small bowl, whisk together the wet ingredients: almond milk, mashed banana (or applesauce), honey (or maple syrup), and melted coconut oil (or butter).
- Pour the wet ingredients into the dry ingredients in the mug and stir until just combined. Do not overmix.
- If using, gently fold in chopped nuts or berries.
- Microwave on high for 45-60 seconds, or until the cake is firm and a toothpick

inserted into the middle comes out clean. Be careful, the mug will be hot!

Cooking Time: 45-60 seconds

Total Preparation Time: 5 minutes

Serving Size: 1

Nutritional Information (approximate per serving):
Calories: 250-300
Protein: 20-25 grams
Carbohydrates: 30-35 grams
Fat: 10-12 grams

<u>**Tips:**</u>

- Experiment with different protein powder flavors to create different cake variations.

- You can use a small amount of cocoa powder for a chocolatey flavor.

- Top your mug cake with a dollop of low-fat Greek yogurt and a sprinkle of berries for extra protein and flavor.

- Make sure your microwave has at least 800 watts. Cooking times may vary according to wattage.

- Let the mug cake cool slightly before digging in, as it will be very hot coming out of the microwave.

Substitutions for Low-Fat Cooking

Strategies for Reducing Fat Content in Recipes:

Here are some clever ways to cut down on the fat content in your favorite recipes without sacrificing flavor:

Swapping Fatty Ingredients:

Fats:

- ***Butter:*** Replace butter with unsweetened applesauce, mashed banana, pureed pumpkin, or low-fat yogurt (depending on the recipe) in a 1:1 ratio. For baking, use canola oil or olive oil in moderation.

- *Cooking Oils:* opt for healthier fats like olive oil, avocado oil, or canola oil. Use them sparingly and avoid deep-frying. Consider using vegetable broth or water for sauteing instead of oil.

- *Cheese:* Choose low-fat or fat-free cheese varieties. Ricotta cheese or cottage cheese can sometimes be used as creamy substitutes in dips and sauces.

Meat:

- *Protein Selection:* Choose lean cuts of meat like skinless chicken breast, turkey breast, lean ground beef, or fish. Trim any visible fat before cooking.

- *Cooking Methods:* Use healthier cooking methods like grilling, baking, roasting, or poaching instead of frying.

Adding Moisture and Flavor:

- *Vegetables:* Add pureed vegetables like roasted red peppers, cauliflower, or zucchini to baked goods for moisture and hidden nutrients.

- *Fruit Purees:* Use unsweetened applesauce, mashed banana, or other fruit purees to add sweetness and moisture to baked goods and pancakes.

- *Broth and Stock:* Utilize low-sodium vegetable broth or chicken broth to add flavor and moisture to soups, stews, and sauces.

- *Herbs and Spices:* Experiment with fresh or dried herbs and spices to create depth of flavor without relying on added fat.

- *Acidity:* A squeeze of lemon juice or vinegar can brighten flavors and sometimes mimic the richness of fat.

- *Non-Stick Cooking Spray:* Use a light coating of non-stick cooking spray to prevent sticking when sauteing or baking.

Recipe Adjustments:

Reduce Overall Fat Content: When following a recipe, try reducing the total amount of fat called for by 25-50%. Often, you won't notice a significant difference in taste or texture.

Portion Control: Be mindful of portion sizes. Even healthy dishes can contribute to weight gain if eaten in excess.

Planning and Preparation:

Read Labels: Pay attention to the fat content of ingredients when grocery shopping. Choose lean cuts of meat, low-fat dairy products, and healthy oils.

Planning Makes Perfect: Plan your meals in advance so you're less likely to reach for unhealthy options when short on time.

Flavorful Alternatives to High-Fat Ingredients:

Here are some specific substitutes you can use to replace high-fat ingredients in your cooking:

High-Fat Ingredient_ Flavorful Alternatives
Butter _ Unsweetened applesauce, mashed banana, pureed pumpkin, low-fat yogurt, olive oil (in moderation)
Cooking Oil_ Vegetable broth, water, non-stick cooking spray

Cream Cheese _	Low-fat ricotta cheese, mashed avocado (in moderation)
Sour Cream_ Low-fat yogurt thinned with milk, low-fat buttermilk.	
Mayonnaise_ Greek yogurt mixed with herbs and spices, mashed avocado (in moderation)	
Heavy Cream_ Low-fat evaporated milk, low-fat milk mixed with cornstarch, cauliflower puree	
Ground Beef_ Lean ground turkey, lentils, chopped mushrooms.	
Whole Milk_ Low-fat milk, skim milk, unsweetened plant-based milk	

By using these strategies and exploring flavorful alternatives, you can enjoy delicious and healthy meals without the extra fat. Remember, a little ingenuity may go a long way in the kitchen!

Effective Meal Planning Strategies for Pancreatitis Diet Success

Let us face it, grocery shopping and meal prep can feel like a never-ending cycle. You battle the crowds, wrestle with overflowing carts, and then spend hours in the kitchen feeling like a short-order cook. But fear not, fellow foodie! I am here to share some tips and tricks that will transform you from a grocery store gladiator into a meal prep master.

Grocery Shopping Strategies

- **Plan Your Battles (Meals):** Before venturing out, plan your meals for the week. Think about what you are craving, what's on sale, and what will fit your busy schedule. This not only saves you money but also prevents those impulse buys that leave you with a fridge full of mystery ingredients and a lighter wallet.

- **Befriend the List (Grocery List):** Make a detailed grocery list, including everything you need for your planned meals, plus some healthy staples like fruits, vegetables, and whole grains. This is your weapon against the siren song of tempting treats!

- **Become a Scouting Pro (Check the Flyers):** Scout out weekly flyers and online coupons before you head to the store. Knowing what's on sale allows you to build your meals around those deals and stretch your grocery budget further.

- **Embrace the Efficiency (Store Layout):** Familiarize yourself with the store layout. Knowing where things are will save you precious time wandering the aisles like a lost soul.

Shopping List Tailored for Meal Prep Success:

Here are sample shopping list to get you started:

- *Proteins:* Choose lean options like chicken breast, salmon, ground turkey, tofu, and lentils.

- *Carbohydrates:* Stock up on brown rice, quinoa, whole-wheat pasta, sweet potatoes, and whole-wheat bread.

- *Vegetables:* Grab a rainbow! Aim for a variety of colorful vegetables like broccoli, carrots, bell peppers, spinach, and leafy greens.

- *Fruits:* Fresh or frozen, fruits are your friends! Berries, bananas, apples, and oranges are all great choices.

- *Healthy Fats:* Keep a healthy oil (like olive oil) and avocados on hand for cooking and adding richness.

- *Seasonings:* Spices and herbs are flavor powerhouses. Stock up on your favorites to keep things interesting.

- *Pantry Staples:* Keep a well-stocked pantry with items like canned beans, whole-wheat pasta sauce, and low-sodium broths for quick meal prep options.

Meal Prep Techniques

- *Batch Cooking is Your Friend:* Cook large batches of protein sources (like grilled chicken or baked salmon) on the weekend. This will save you time throughout the week for assembling meals.

- **Chop Like a Ninja:** Dedicate some time on the weekend to chopping vegetables. This will make assembling meals throughout the week a breeze.

- **Portion Control is Key:** Portion out your meals into containers for the week. This helps avoid overeating and ensures you have healthy, pre-made meals readily available when hunger strikes.

- **Get Creative with Leftovers:** Leftovers don't have to be boring! Repurpose them into new dishes. For example, leftover roasted chicken can be chopped and added to salads, wraps, or pasta dishes.

- **Embrace the Freezer:** Certain prepped items like cooked quinoa, chopped vegetables, and cooked ground meat can be frozen for later use. This is a lifesaver on those extra-busy weeks.

Remember, meal prep is about making your life easier and healthier. Do not be scared to explore and discover what works best for you. With a little planning and these handy tips, you will be a grocery shopping and meal prep pro in no time! *Now go forth and conquer that kitchen!*

Balance meal plan for pancreatitis with perfect timing to consume.

Week 1:

Day 1:

Breakfast (7:00 AM): High-Protein Smoothie (energizing start)
Lunch (12:30 PM): Chicken Caesar Salad with Grilled Chicken Breast, Protein Powder (light and satisfying)
Dinner (7:00 PM): Baked Cod with Lemon and Herbs, Quinoa (flavorful and protein-rich)
Snacks (choose 2 throughout the day):
10:00 AM: Edamame pods with chili flakes
4:00 PM: Cottage Cheese with Sliced Bell Peppers
Brunch Option (10:00 AM): Türkiye and Veggie Frittata (enjoy a leisurely weekend brunch)

Day 2:

Breakfast (7:30 AM): Tofu Scramble with Turkey Sausage (savory and protein-packed)
Lunch (1:00 PM): Lentil and Black Bean Salad with Quinoa (hearty and filling)
Dinner (7:30 PM): Turkey Breast with Brown Rice and Steamed Broccoli (classic and comforting)
Snacks (choose 2 throughout the day):
11:00 AM: Homemade trail mix
3:00 PM: Greek yogurt topped with berries and protein powder.

Day 3:

Breakfast (8:00 AM): Egg White Frittata with Vegetables (versatile and customizable)
Lunch (12:00 PM): Turkey Burger on Whole-Wheat Bun with Avocado (moderation) (satisfying and flavorful)
Dinner (6:30 PM): Shrimp and Vegetable Curry with Quinoa (exotic and nutritious)
Snacks (choose 2 throughout the day):

2:00 PM: Hard-boiled Eggs with Cottage Cheese
5:00 PM: Roasted Chickpeas with Spices
Brunch Option (10:30 AM): Shrimp and Quinoa Salad with Avocado (moderation) (lighter brunch)

Day 4:

Breakfast (7:00 AM): Chicken Sausage and Veggie Muffins (grab-and-go convenience)
Lunch (1:00 PM): Tuna Salad Sandwich with Cottage Cheese on Whole-Wheat Bread (light and protein-rich)
Dinner (7:00 PM): Tofu Veggie Burgers on Whole-Wheat Buns with Sweet Potato Fries (fun and satisfying)
Snacks (choose 2 throughout the day):
9:00 AM: Sliced turkey breast with cucumber slices
4:00 PM: Air-popped popcorn with nutritional yeast

Day 5:

Breakfast (8:00 AM): Greek Yogurt Parfait with Nuts and Seeds (creamy and delicious)

Lunch (12:30 PM): Shrimp Scampi with Whole-Wheat Pasta and Asparagus (light and elegant)
Dinner (7:00 PM): Chicken and Vegetable Kabobs with Brown Rice (a colorful and protein-rich option)
Snacks (choose 2 throughout the day):
10:00 AM: High-Protein Smoothie
3:00 PM: Baked Chicken Breast Strips with yogurt dip
Brunch Option (11:00 AM): Salmon with Roasted Sweet Potatoes and Asparagus (hearty weekend brunch)

Day 6:

Breakfast (7:30 AM): High-Protein Oatmeal with Berries (warm and satisfying)
Lunch (1:00 PM): Lentil Soup with Cottage Cheese (comforting and light)
Dinner (6:00 PM): Lentil Shepherd's Pie with Protein-Fortified Mashed Potatoes (a hearty and comforting classic)

> **Snacks (choose 2 throughout the day):** Leftover fruits or vegetables from the week (anytime)

Day 7:

> **Breakfast (8:00 AM):** Scrambled Eggs with Black Beans and Salsa (savory and protein-packed)

> **Lunch (12:00 PM):** Chickpea Salad Pita with Vegetables (portable and refreshing)

> **Dinner (7:00 PM):** Baked Salmon with Roasted Brussels Sprouts and Quinoa (another delicious salmon option)

> **Snacks (choose 2 throughout the day):** Pick your favorites from the week.

Week 2:

Day 8:

> **Breakfast (7:00 AM):** Protein Smoothie Bowl (a refreshing and energizing start)

> **Lunch (1:00 PM):** Tofu and Veggie Stir-Fry with Quinoa (light and flavorful)

Dinner (7:30 PM): Flank Steak Fajitas with Whole-Wheat Tortillas (fun and interactive)
Snacks (choose 2 throughout the day):
10:00 AM: Edamame pods with chili flakes
4:00 PM: Cottage Cheese with Sliced Bell Peppers
Brunch Option (10:30 AM): Tofu Scramble Breakfast Burrito (enjoy a protein-packed weekend brunch)

Day 9:

Breakfast (7:30 AM): Chicken Breast with Whole-Wheat Pancakes and Berries (satisfying and sweet)
Lunch (12:30 PM): Salmon with Quinoa Salad (light and protein-rich)
Dinner (6:30 PM): Shrimp and Asparagus Stir-Fry with Brown Rice (quick and flavorful)
Snacks (choose 2 throughout the day):
11:00 AM: Homemade trail mix
3:00 PM: Greek yogurt with protein powder and berries

Day 10:

Breakfast (8:00 AM): Turkey Bacon and Whole-Wheat Pancakes (classic and satisfying)
Lunch (1:00 PM): High-Protein Chicken Soup with Brown Rice (comforting and light)
Dinner (7:00 PM): Chicken Breast with Quinoa and Roasted Vegetables (a balanced and colorful option)
Snacks (choose 2 throughout the day):
10:00 AM: Hard-boiled Eggs with Cottage Cheese
3:00 PM: Roasted Chickpeas with Spices

Day 11:

Breakfast (7:00 AM): Baked Apples with Cinnamon and Protein Powder (approved by your doctor) (warm and sweet)
Lunch (12:30 PM): Turkey and Vegetable Wrap with Cottage Cheese (portable and protein-rich)
Dinner (7:00 PM): Baked Cod with Lemon and Herbs, Quinoa (flavorful and protein-rich)
Snacks (choose 2 throughout the day):
9:00 AM: Sliced turkey breast with cucumber slices

4:00 PM: Air-popped popcorn with nutritional yeast

Day 12:

Breakfast (8:00 AM): High-Protein Yogurt Parfait (creamy and delicious)
Lunch (1:00 PM): Tuna Salad Sandwich with Cottage Cheese on Whole-Wheat Bread (light and protein-rich)
Dinner (7:30 PM): Turkey Breast with Brown Rice and Steamed Broccoli (classic and comforting)
Snacks (choose 2 throughout the day):
10:00 AM: High-Protein Smoothie (energizing)
3:00 PM: Baked Chicken Breast Strips with yogurt dip
Brunch Option (11:00 AM): Chicken Sausage and Veggie Muffins (grab-and-go convenience)

Day 13:

Breakfast (7:30 AM): Scrambled Eggs with Black Beans and Salsa (savory and protein-packed)
Lunch (12:00 PM): Lentil and Black Bean Salad with Quinoa (hearty and filling)
Dinner (6:00 PM): Shrimp and Vegetable Curry with Quinoa (exotic and nutritious)
Snacks (choose 2 throughout the day): Leftover fruits or vegetables from the week (anytime)

Day 14:

Breakfast (8:00 AM): Egg White Frittata with Vegetables (versatile and customizable)
Lunch (1:00 PM): Chickpea Salad Pita with Vegetables (portable and refreshing)
Dinner (7:00 PM): Lentil Shepherd's Pie with Protein-Fortified Mashed Potatoes (a hearty and comforting classic)
Snacks (choose 2 throughout the day): Pick your favorites from the week (anytime)

Week 3:

Day 15:

Breakfast (7:00 AM): Protein Smoothie Bowl (a refreshing and energizing start)
Lunch (1:00 PM): Chicken Caesar Salad with Grilled Chicken Breast, Protein Powder (light and satisfying)
Dinner (7:30 PM): Tofu Veggie Burgers on Whole-Wheat Buns with Sweet Potato Fries (fun and satisfying)
Snacks (choose 2 throughout the day):
10:00 AM: Cottage Cheese with Sliced Bell Peppers
4:00 PM: Homemade trail mix
Brunch Option (10:30 AM): Salmon with Roasted Sweet Potatoes and Asparagus (hearty weekend brunch)

Day 16:

Breakfast (7:30 AM): Tofu Scramble with Turkey Sausage (savory and protein-packed)

Lunch (12:30 PM): Shrimp Scampi with Whole-Wheat Pasta and Asparagus (light and elegant)
Dinner (6:30 PM): Chicken and Vegetable Kabobs with Brown Rice (a colorful and protein-rich option)
Snacks (choose 2 throughout the day):
11:00 AM: Greek yogurt with protein powder and berries
3:00 PM: Hard-boiled Eggs with Cottage Cheese

Day 17:

Breakfast (8:00 AM): High-Protein Oatmeal with Berries (warm and satisfying)
Lunch (1:00 PM): Turkey Burger on Whole-Wheat Bun with Avocado (moderation) (satisfying and flavorful)
Dinner (7:00 PM): Baked Salmon with Roasted Brussels Sprouts and Quinoa (another delicious salmon option)
Snacks (choose 2 throughout the day):
10:00 AM: Edamame pods with chili flakes
3:00 PM: Sliced turkey breast with cucumber slices

Day 18:

Breakfast (7:00 AM): Greek Yogurt Parfait with Nuts and Seeds (creamy and delicious)
Lunch (12:30 PM): Tofu and Veggie Stir-Fry with Quinoa (light and flavorful)
Dinner (7:00 PM): Flank Steak Fajitas with Whole-Wheat Tortillas (fun and interactive
Snacks (choose 2 throughout the day):
9:00 AM: Air-popped popcorn with nutritional yeast
4:00 PM: Roasted Chickpeas with Spices
Brunch Option (11:00 AM): Chicken Breast with Whole-Wheat Pancakes and Berries (satisfying and sweet)

Day 19:

Breakfast (8:00 AM): Chicken Sausage and Veggie Muffins (grab-and-go convenience
Lunch (1:00 PM): Lentil Soup with Cottage Cheese (comforting and light)
Dinner (7:30 PM): Shrimp and Asparagus Stir-Fry with Brown Rice (quick and flavorful)

Snacks (choose 2 throughout the day):
10:00 AM: High-Protein Smoothie
3:00 PM: Baked Apples with Cinnamon and Protein Powder

Day 20:

Breakfast (7:30 AM): Türkiye Bacon and Whole-Wheat Pancakes (classic and satisfying)
Lunch (12:00 PM): Salmon with Quinoa Salad (light and protein-rich)
Dinner (6:00 PM): Chicken Breast with Quinoa and Roasted Vegetables

Day 21:

Breakfast (8:00 AM): Scrambled Eggs with Black Beans and Salsa (savory and protein-packed)
Lunch (1:00 PM): Chickpea Salad Pita with Vegetables (portable and refreshing)
Dinner (7:00 PM): Baked Cod with Lemon and Herbs, Quinoa (flavorful and protein-rich) (repeat from Week 1)

Snacks (choose 2 throughout the day): Pick your favorites from the week (anytime)
Desserts (throughout the 3 weeks):

Feel free to indulge in any of the dessert options (Baked apples with cinnamon, High-Protein Yogurt Parfait, Frozen Greek Yogurt with Berries, Chia Seed Pudding, or Protein Mug Cake) on occasion, but remember to practice moderation!

Remember:

This is a guideline. Feel free to adjust portion sizes, swap recipes, and timings based on your preferences and schedule.

Utilize leftovers creatively to minimize food waste and maximize variety.

For optimum health, sip water often throughout the day.

Most importantly, enjoy the delicious and nutritious meals!

Cooking Techniques for Gentle Pancreatic Support

Cooking Like a Nutrient Ninja

Ever wonder how to whip up delicious meals that tantalize your taste buds while keeping your body happy? The answer lies in smart cooking methods! Let us explore some techniques that help preserve the nutrients in your food and aid digestion, making you feel fantastic from the inside out.

Cooking Methods that Preserve Nutrients and Aid Digestion:

- **Steaming:** Think of steaming as a gentle kiss for your veggies. It uses steam to cook food without submerging it in water, which can leach out valuable vitamins and minerals. Imagine crisp broccoli florets or fluffy fish filets retaining their vibrant colors and delicate flavors – a visual and taste bud treat! Plus, steaming is easy on your digestive system, making it a perfect choice for anyone with a sensitive tummy.

- **Roasting:** Roasting is like giving your food a warm hug in the oven. It brings out the natural sweetness of vegetables and caramelizes proteins on meats, creating a delightful depth of flavor. Imagine the aroma of roasted rosemary chicken or golden brown sweet potatoes filling your kitchen – pure comfort food magic! The dry heat of roasting also helps retain nutrients and allows for minimal added fat, keeping things light and healthy.

- **Poaching:** Poaching is a gentle simmering technique, often used for eggs and fish. Imagine perfectly cooked eggs with runny yolks or delicate fish flakes – a culinary masterpiece! This method is a champion for nutrient preservation and cooks food so gently that it's easily digestible, making it a great choice for anyone looking for a lighter option.

- **Stir-frying:** Stir-frying is a quick and vibrant cooking method that uses minimal oil. Imagine colorful veggies and lean protein coming together in a symphony of flavors and textures – a visual and taste bud party! The high heat and short cooking time help retain nutrients, while the minimal oil keeps things light and healthy. Plus, stir-frying is a fantastic way to incorporate a variety of veggies into your meals, boosting your intake of essential vitamins and minerals.

Tips for Tenderizing Foods Without Excess Fat:

Marinating: Marinating is like giving your food a flavorful bath! Soaking meats, poultry, or even tofu in a marinade packed with herbs, spices, and acids (like lemon juice or vinegar) helps break down tough fibers, resulting in incredibly tender and flavorful bites. Imagine juicy, melt-in-your-mouth chicken or perfectly cooked tofu – a textural delight! Marinating not only tenderizes but also infuses your food with delicious flavors, reducing the need for added salt or unhealthy fats.

Slow Cooking: Embrace the magic of slow cooking! This method uses low heat and a long cooking time to gently break down tough fibers, resulting in fall-off-the-bone goodness. Imagine a pot roast so tender it practically melts in your mouth – pure comfort food heaven! Slow cooking allows the natural flavors of your ingredients to develop beautifully, and the low heat helps preserve nutrients.

Mechanical Tenderizing: Sometimes, a little physical persuasion goes a long way. Techniques like pounding with a meat mallet or using a meat tenderizer can help break down tough fibers in meats, making them chewier and easier to digest. Imagine perfectly cooked steaks or juicy burgers – a carnivore's dream! Just remember, don't overdo it, or you might end up with mushy meat. By incorporating these techniques into your cooking repertoire, you will be well on your way to creating delicious and nutritious meals that nourish your body and taste buds. Remember, cooking should be a fun and rewarding experience. So, experiment, get creative, and enjoy the journey to becoming a nutrient ninja in the kitchen!

Conclusion

This comprehensive guide has equipped you with the knowledge and tools to navigate your pancreatic journey with confidence. We have explored a variety of delicious and nutritious meal plans, cooking methods that preserve nutrients, and tips for gentle food preparation. You've learned how to listen to your body's hunger cues and space out meals for optimal digestion.

Key Points to Remember:

Food is Medicine: The right diet plays a vital role in managing pancreatitis and promoting long-term pancreatic health. Embrace the variety of delicious and nourishing recipes offered in this guide.

Listen to Your Body: Pay attention to your body's hunger cues and adjust meal schedules accordingly. Try out different things until you find what works best for you.

Small and Frequent Wins: opt for smaller, more frequent meals to promote better digestion and help maintain consistent blood sugar levels.

Embrace the Kitchen: Do not be intimidated by cooking! Utilize the tips and techniques explored in this guide to create healthy and flavorful meals you will genuinely enjoy.

Remember, managing pancreatitis is a journey, not a destination. There will be bumps along the road, but with the knowledge and tools you have gained, you're empowered to make informed decisions and prioritize your well-being. Celebrate your small victories as you navigate this journey. Every healthy choice you make is a step towards a healthier and happier you.

Most importantly, do not hesitate to seek support from your healthcare team. They are there to guide you and ensure you have a successful and empowering pancreatic journey. With the right tools and unwavering determination, you can thrive on your path to optimal health.

Milton Keynes UK
Ingram Content Group UK Ltd.
UKHW021406181124
2928UKWH00070B/1981

9 798321 606070